Healing Power of FOODS

Nature's Prescriptions for Common Diseases

Sunita Pant Bansal

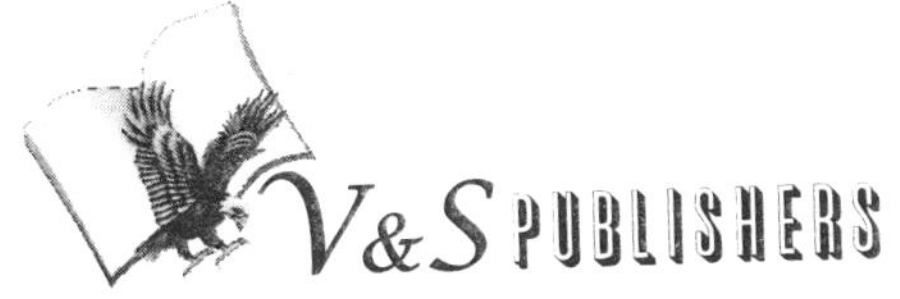

Published by:

F-2/16, Ansari Road, Daryaganj, New Delhi-110002
☎ 011-23240026, 011-23240027 • *Fax* 011-23240028
Email info@vspublishers.com • *Website* www.vspublishers.com

Regional Office Hyderabad
5-1-707/1, Brij Bhawan (Beside Central Bank of India Lane)
Bank Street, Koti, Hyderabad - 500 095
☎ 040-24737290
E-mail vspublishershyd@gmail.com

Branch Office : Mumbai
Jaywant Industrial Estate, 1st Floor–108, Tardeo Road
Opposite Sobo Central Mall, Mumbai – 400 034
☎ 022-23510736
E-mail: vspublishersmum@gmail.com

Follow us on: 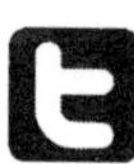 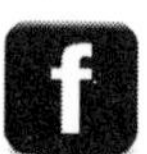 

All books available at **www.vspublishers.com**

ISBN 978-93-813842-3-7

Edition: 2019

Printed at : Param Offseters, Okhla, New Delhi-110020

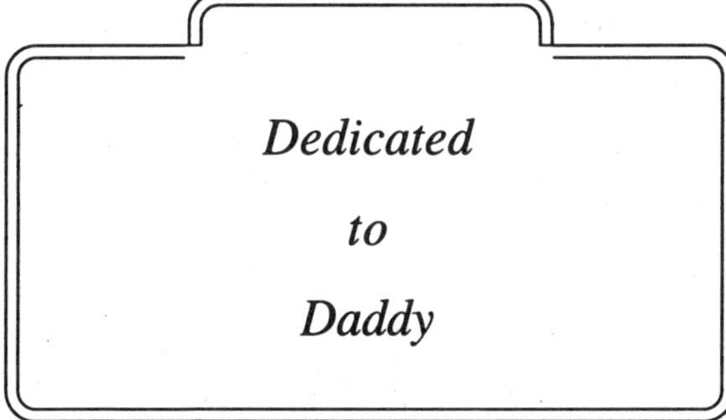
Dedicated
to
Daddy

ACKNOWLEDGEMENT

This book is dedicated to my father, who instilled the importance of nutrition in my life. Had he lived, I am sure he would have been very proud of the way my hundreds of articles on food and nutrition have culminated into this book.

Words cannot express my feelings of gratitude towards the two most important people in my life, without whose constant encouragement and support; I would not have been what I am today. They are, my mother and my husband.

Thanks are due to my friend Shruti Sharma, who helped me in data collection and to Vandana Arya and Alex Tom for deciphering my handwriting and typing the manuscript.

—Sunita Pant Bansal
NOIDA, (U.P.)

Contents

INTRODUCTION

A significant percentage of people have preventable disorders, many of which are caused by routine violations of good health and nutritional habits. Even borderline deficiencies can lead to different types of illnesses.

Insufficient or inaccurate knowledge, inability to obtain nutritious foodstuffs and supplements, and/or indifferent attitude towards self-care are the most common underlying reasons behind poor eating habits and resulting sickness. For example, all substances consumed in excess are toxic to the body. Consuming the same foods day after day, saturate the body and intoxicate it. Ultimately, rather than nourishing these foods repeatedly cause the body to react negatively. Even today most people believe that diet is only important in relation to weight loss and bodybuilding. Whereas, the diet is an important factor in overall health and well-being.

The right foods do have the power to heal just as the wrong foods can cause ill health. In India, Ayurveda has been around for many centuries. People not knowing Ayurveda have also been using indigenous herbs/ plants as household remedies since times immemorial, especially in villages and small towns, where access to medical facilities is not easy. Not only in India, herbs and plant food therapy has been successful through the ages all over the world. Why? Because the plants have certain properties that cure the disease and restore the natural balance in the body.

The drug industry has isolated the key components from the plants to use in the various therapies. For example, the most powerful drug used in cancer chemotherapy was isolated from the plant Madagascar Periwinkle. It is effective against breast cancer, but its side effects may be debilitating. Nature intended all the parts of the plant to work together, as buffers and regulators, minimizing side effects and aiding assimilation.

This book is an attempt to make available nature's pharmacopoeia to the readers, as it is essential to know which plant/herb has therapeutic applications in which disorder/disease.

VEGETABLES

People have this misconception that a nutritious diet necessarily involves the use of expensive food articles. They forget that nature also provides us with food articles that are nutritious and can be obtained at a relatively low cost. Unfortunately, there exist some hurdles in the way of use of the vegetables. Often people are influenced by the traditional food taboos and beliefs that have no scientific basis. This is further complicated by the fact that people are carried away by the status value attached to a food unmindful of its nutritive value. For instance, it is a common belief that green leafy vegetables are poor man's food and that it is not prestigious to consume them. It is true that the leaves are inexpensive, however, this does not make them in any way inferior in their nutritive value.

Now let us see these vegetables with a different eye- the eye of a nutritionist. After all, what do these vegetables provide? All vegetables have one thing in common; they provide little energy and more of vitamins and mineral than any other food item.

Green leafy vegetables in general are rich in iron, calcium, vitamins A and C. Iron is required for the formation of haemoglobin (the red factor) in the blood, and vitamin C enhances the absorption of iron by our body system. They are also good for the eyes because of their good vitamin A content.

All the red and yellow vegetables like tomatoes and pumpkin are rich in vitamin A. Other vegetables like brinjal, bitter gourds are rich in B group vitamins. Other than vitamins, the vegetables also have good amounts of minerals like iron, potassium and calcium and of course fibre.

Vegetables are useful in weight reducing diets, as they provide bulk and give a feeling of satiety but provide few calories. The bulk and water content of vegetables also helps in the treatment of constipation.

There is a misconception that vegetables produce diarrhoea, especially in small children. This is a wrong notion. The fact is that the vegetables, especially the leafy contain large amounts of dirt and germs, which if not cleaned, will certainly produce diarrhoea. So they should be carefully washed before using.

In order to get the best out of the vegetables, they should be preferably used fresh and washed thoroughly before they are cut. The vessel in which they are cooked should be covered with a lid to prevent the loss of vitamin C. Frying and drying in the sun results in some carotene (vitamin A) loss, but do not be disheartened, other important nutrients like iron remain safe.

Vegetables should be consumed daily in diet in some form or the other - as vegetable dishes, cooked with dal or as salad. Other than maintaining good health, the vegetables also have curative powers, a fact which has been proved many times in many ailments including cancer.

AMARANTH (*Chaulai*)

Amaranth is the most common leafy vegetable grown during the summer in India. The leaves and tender stems are rich in vitamins A, B and C.

Amaranth contains minerals like magnesium, phosphorus, sodium, calcium, iron, potassium and sulphur in appreciable amounts.

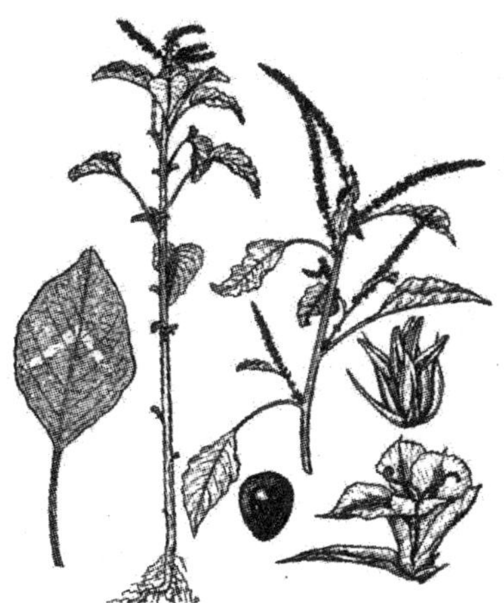

As Meaicine:

- The juice of amaranth leaves is effective in resolving cataract.
- Boiled leaves taken regularly can cure night blindness.

BITTER GOURD (*Karela*)

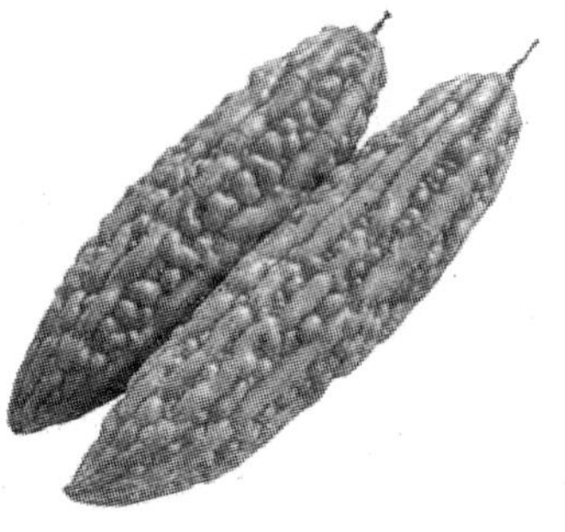

Bitter gourd is a unique vegetable in the sense, that it is coveted by many because of its bitter taste.

It is a very nutritious vegetable, the smaller the size, the more nutrients it seems to contain. It is an excellent source of vitamin C and contains most of the B complex vitamins, and vitamin A (in the form of carotene) too. It also has calcium, phosphorus, potassium and iron in appreciable amounts.

As Medicine:

- The bitter principle of karela is found in all the parts of the plant, and is considered to be wormicidal and generally good for stomach disorders.
- In the autumn and spring seasons, boiled bitter gourd should be eaten as a preventive against chicken pox and measles.
- For disorders of spleen and liver, bitter gourd extract is considered beneficial.
- For diabetes, a mixture of equal quantities of amla juice and bitter gourd juice taken every morning show a reduction in blood glucose levels.
- The leaves are said to increase the milk production in lactating mothers.
- For bleeding piles and intestinal worms, juice extracted from bitter gourd leaves mixed with buttermilk is prescribed.
- Dried and powdered bitter gourd leaves are applied locally on burns, boils and other skin eruptions.

BEETROOT (*Chukandar*)

This fleshy root vegetable is popular as a salad item. It is rich in iron, potassium, calcium and vitamins A and C.

Beets are not only good for the eliminative system, but also benefit the digestive and lymphatic systems. They offer an excellent remedy for anaemia, general debility, low vitality, lassitude and nervous debility.

They may be eaten raw or taken in the form of juice.

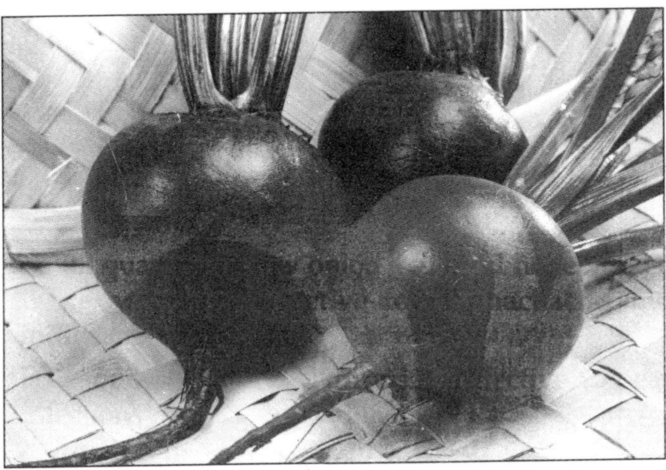

As Medicine:

- Beet juice is one of the most valuable juices for the liver and gall bladder.
- The root is rich in iron and helps in the generation of red blood cells in anaemia.
- Raw beetroot is prescribed in cancer as it has a tumour-inhibiting component.

BRINJAL (*Baigan*)

Brinjal or eggplant is available in plenty when other fresh vegetables are scarce.

Brinjals contain higher amounts of vitamin B than other vegetables. Dark purple coloured brinjals have a good vitamin C content–better than the light coloured ones. All brinjals are rich in minerals, especially magnesium and potassium, good for muscle tone and strength.

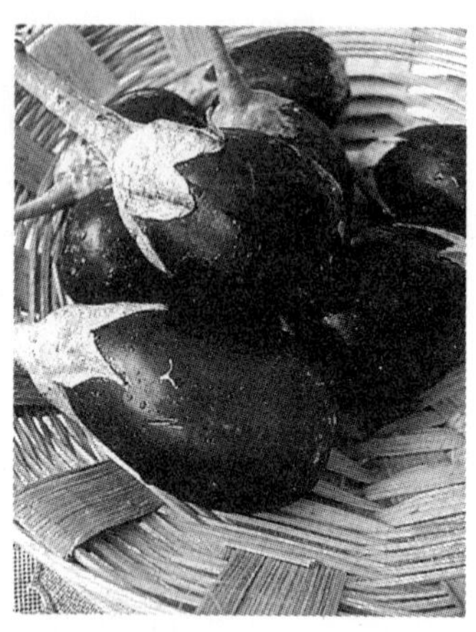

As Medicine:

- The roots of this plant are known to be anti-asthmatic.
- The leaves have narcotic property, forming a base for many medicines.
- Both the leaves and the fruit of brinjal are reported to produce a marked drop in the blood cholesterol levels.
- Brinjal juice is found to be an effective remedy for toothache.

BOTTLE GOURD (*Lauki*)

It is extensively grown in India. The fruits in the green stage are used as vegetables and also for preparation of some sweets. The hard shell of the fruit has many uses. They are used as water jugs, domestic utensils, making musical instruments, floats for fishing nets and many other purposes.

Bottle gourd contains vitamins A, B and C, iron, magnesium, sodium, potassium, sulphur and fibre.

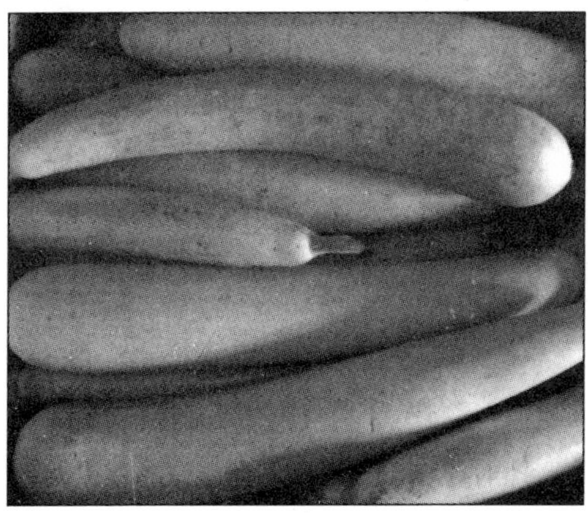

As Medicine:

- The pulp and the young stem and leaves have many medicinal values. Their extract is used to relieve earache and the pulp used as poultice on the eyes relieves eyestrain and pain.
- The bitter fruits are poisonous and are used as a strong purgative.

CABBAGE (*Patta Gobhi*)

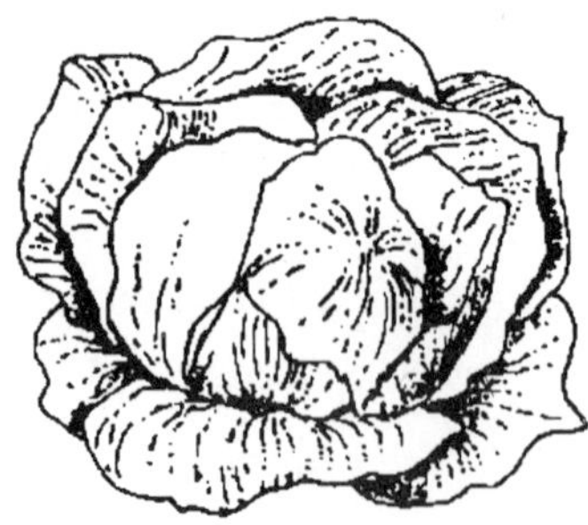

Cabbage is one of the healthiest vegetables. Cabbage is alkaline in reaction, high in cellulose or roughage, and has a very low calorie content. It stabilizes chemical reactions in the body. It is excellent as a vitalizing agent, and a blood purifier.

Cabbage contains many minerals: it is rich in calcium and potassium, and contains iodine, phosphorus, sodium, and sulphur.

It is an excellent source of vitamins A, B and C.

As Medicine:

- It is prescribed in cases of afternoon headaches, listlessness, depression, palpitation, neuralgia, bronchitis and jaundice.
- The use of cabbage juice for treatment of stomach ulcers is one of the latest and most vital advances in the field of juice therapy.
- It is also used in the treatment of colon cancer. The juice inhibits the growth of tumours and heals the inflammation of the colon and stomach.
- Applying cabbage paste helps eczema and other skin infections to clear.
- Cabbage is therapeutically effective in conditions of scurvy, goitre, diseases of the eyes, gout, rheumatism and pyorrhoea.
- Cabbage is very effective in helping overcome constipation.
- Cabbage is considered one of the best foods for keeping a clean, clear complexion.

CARROT (*Gaajar*)

Carrot is a very popular vegetable in the Indian cuisine, both raw as well as cooked. Besides containing iron, calcium and phosphorus, carrots contain appreciable amounts of beta-carotene, which the body converts into vitamin A. These carotenids have been linked to the prevention of certain types of cancer, particularly lung cancer.

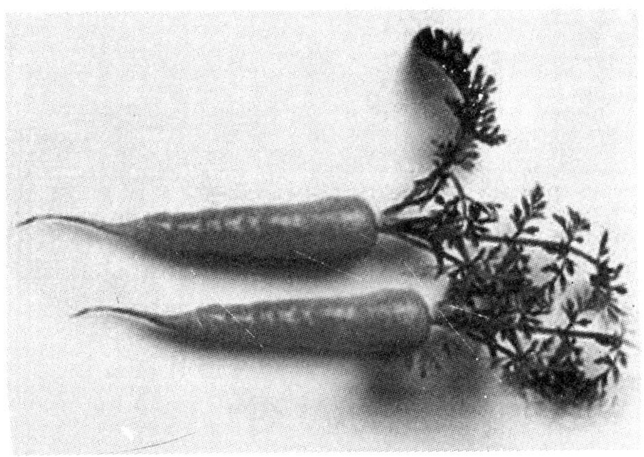

Carrots are rich in fibre. A high fibre does not only help in lowering blood sugar and cholesterol levels but also helps in preventing cancer of the intestine especially the large intestine.

The best way to absorb nutrients from carrots is to eat them raw. If cooked, quite a bit of the nutrients are lost. If stored at very low temperatures (frozen), carrots retain their nutritive value even till 5 or 6 months.

As Medicine:

- A cup of carrot juice taken daily improves the eyesight and prevents cataract.
- Many children have lower jaws that are underdeveloped. This deformity is usually the result of calcium deficiency in the child's early growth.

It is good for a child to have a raw carrot with each meal. The teeth of children straighten out and the lower jaw develops in a year, when they are given a carrot to chew on before each meal.

- 2 to 3 raw carrots taken daily in the diet help in all cases of constipation, worm infestations and reduce the blood cholesterol.
- Carrot soup and/or fresh juice is excellent for the treatment of infantile diarrhoea, even in newborns, premature infants, and in all children suffering from acute colitis or diarrhoea. It also helps the adults with acute diarrhoea, and all intestinal/colon disorders. Carrot soup also prevents dehydration.
- Carrots along with their leaves, eaten regularly in any form, aid in the treatment and/or prevention of gout and all forms of arthritis, skin disorders, hair loss and cancers.
- Carrot juice with a little honey is highly effective in all sorts of fevers, general debility, nervous disorders, anaemia, lassitude, low vitality, and run-down conditions.
- A poultice of boiled carrots heals sores on any part of the body.
- Carrot juice applied on the burns helps them to heal faster.

CAULIFLOWER (*Phool Gobhi*)

Cauliflower is a member of the cabbage family and has similar properties. Cauliflower contains compounds that stimulate the natural defences to neutralize carcinogens. It is high in essential sulphur compounds. Cauliflower is also rich in vitamin C, potassium and fibre. This vegetable is better than cabbage for diabetic people.

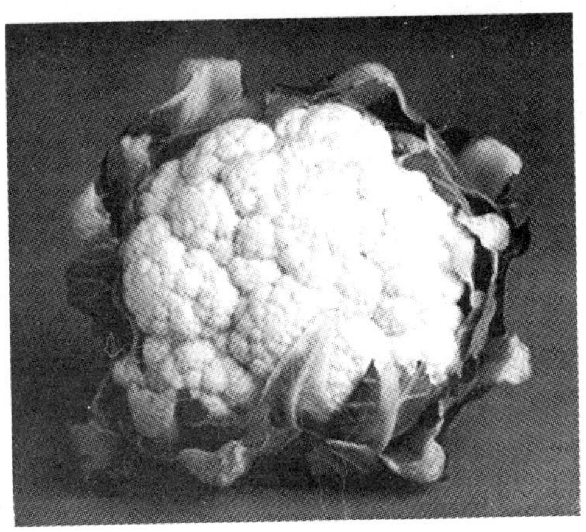

As Medicine:

- Use the cauliflower leaves as cooked or as salad. The greatest amount of calcium in cauliflower is found in the greens that are around the head.
- Regular intake of cauliflower reduces the risk of cancer, particularly of the colon, rectum and stomach and possibly the prostate.
- Cauliflower is also good for reducing diets, because it is low in calories.

CUCUMBER (*Kheera*)

It is a favourite vegetable during hot summer months as it keeps the body cool. It prevents sunstroke and/or heat stroke and quenches thirst. Cucumbers are wonderful as a digestive aid, and have a purifying effect on the bowel. They have a marvellous effect on the skin.

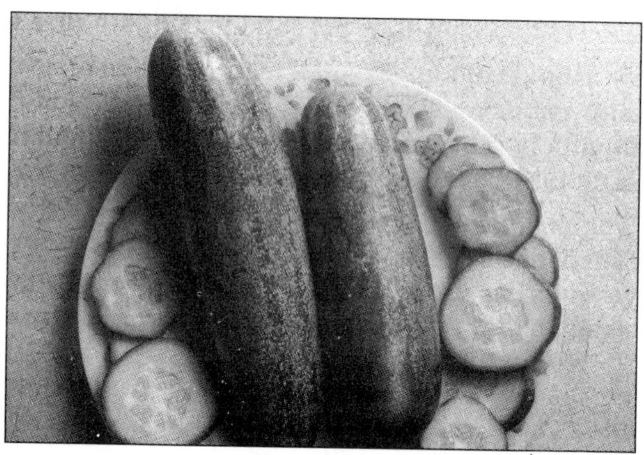

As Medicine:

- Slices of cucumber are used to draw out the poison from an insect bite.
- Slices or poultice of crushed cucumber are good for tired and puffy eyes.
- Cucumber promotes urination, is good for the spleen, stomach and large intestine.
- It is also an effective blood cleanser, hence good for acne and general health of the skin.
- A daily intake of cucumber, along with its peel, prevents kidney stones.

CORIANDER (*Dhania*)

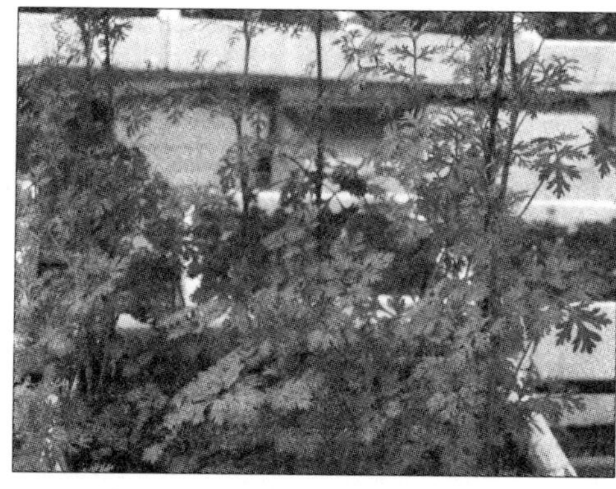

A most popular garnish, especially in Indian recipes. Coriander leaves are not only good for beautifying the dishes but also neutralize gastric acidity. Coriander-mint chutney is a favourite meal accompaniment, having appetizing as well as carminative properties. The seeds as well as the leaves kill bacteria and fungi and are good for anyone who has gastritis and other symptoms of acidity.

As Medicine:

- Dysentery, hepatitis, indigestion, nausea: 1 to 2 tsp fresh juice of coriander leaves mixed in 1 teacup buttermilk to be taken 2-3 times daily.
- Haemorrhoids: Equal quantities of ground coriander leaves and red clay mixed into a fine paste to be applied on the affected part at bedtime helps the Haemorrhoids to heal.
- Bleeding nose: Juice of fresh coriander leaves can be used as nasal drops.
- Blackheads, pimples: One teaspoon turmeric powder made into a paste with juice of fresh coriander leaves, and applied daily as a face pack before going to bed.
- Rashes on the skin: Coriander leaf paste applied on the affected area helps.

DRUMSTICK (*Saijan*)

The pods of drumstick are mostly used in the south Indian cuisine. The special flavour of sambhar is due to this vegetable. Drumsticks have appreciable amounts of calcium, iron, phosphorus and vitamin C. They are also rich in facilitators like, folic acid, which helps in the absorption of iron; and beta-carotene, which helps in the synthesis of vitamin A.

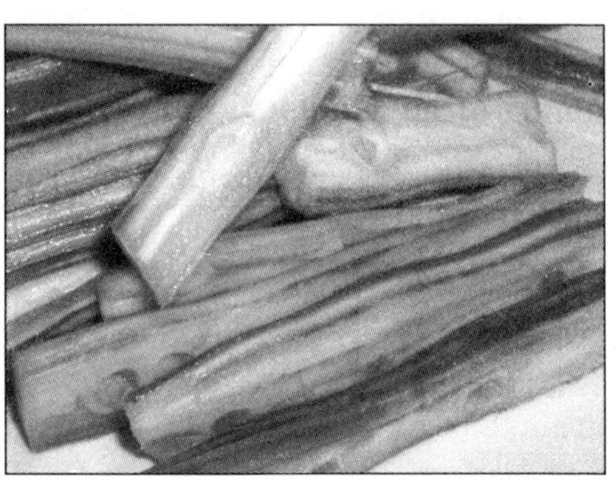

As Medicine:

- A fine paste of the drumstick bark applied daily on the bald patches, promote hair growth.
- Equal quantities of limejuice and the juice of the fresh leaves of the drumstick plant applied on the blackheads and pimples regularly, help in getting rid of them.
- Soup of equal quantities of drumstick and carrots boiled together, is good for lowering blood pressure.
- Regular intake of drumsticks helps in the prevention of joint pains and chronic fatigue.

FENUGREEK (*Methi*)

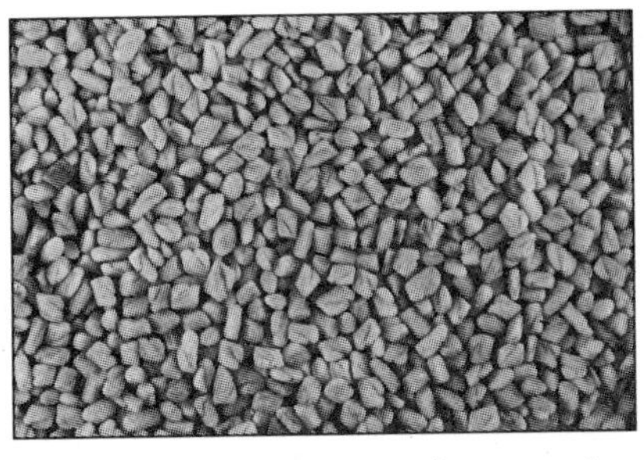

Methi seeds as well as leaves are an important part of Indian cooking. Both help in cooling down the body, reducing mucous in sinus and asthmatic conditions. They soothe down persistent coughs and lower cholesterol. The seeds make excellent tea for intestinal inflammation and irritation and as a gargle tea for sore throats.

As Medicine:

- Skin-irritations, sores, tumours and wounds: Leaves cooked with coconut milk, to be taken once a day for 2-3 days.
- Biliousness, stomach problem: Boiled fenugreek leaves to be eaten twice daily.
- Headache and insomnia: 2 tsp fresh juice of fenugreek leaves along with 1 tsp honey to be taken daily.
- Constipation, duodenal ulcers: Boiled leaves with honey twice daily.
- Falling hair, dullness and coarseness of hair: Fresh leaf paste applied over scalp before bath.
- Mouth ulcers, sore throat: An infusion of leaves gargled 5-6 times daily for a couple of days.
- Blackheads, wrinkles and pimples: Fresh leaf paste applied on face every night before going to bed and washed off with warm water next morning.
- Boils, swellings: Lukewarm leaf paste to be applied on the affected parts of the body.

GARLIC (*Lahsun*)

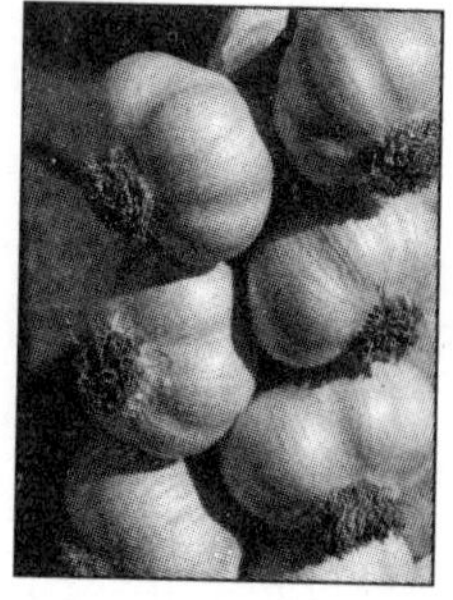

Garlic has been held in high esteem for its medicinal use for centuries. It is an effective detoxifier of blood and lymph in the body. It dilates the peripheral blood vessels, resulting in lowering the blood pressure.

Garlic is high in iodine and sulphur, hence good for goitre. It has a favourable effect on the mucous membrane of the throat and the air passages of the lungs, and is extremely helpful in cases of asthma and hay fever.

It is one of the most powerful natural antibiotics and antiseptics known to man. Garlic cures intestinal and lung disorders, worms, skin diseases, wounds and slows down ageing.

As Medicine:

- Arteriosclerosis, hypertension and bronchial catarrh: 3 cloves of garlic, chopped and boiled in milk and taken every night.
- High blood sugar, high cholesterol: Regular intake of garlic cloves for a few days.
- Severe digestive disorders, dysentery: Take 3 to 6 crushed garlic cloves with honey once or twice a day.
- Intestinal parasites: 3-4 garlic cloves steeped in water or milk overnight; the liquor to be taken the next day.
- Earache: Boil well 1tsp garlic in 2 tbsp oil. Cool and filter. Use as eardrops (2 to 3 drops).
- Cold, phlegm and tropical eosinophilia: 2 garlic cloves crushed, boiled in a cup of water along with ½ tsp turmeric powder.
- Acne, boils, corns in the foot, warts, etc.: Mash the garlic cloves and apply externally.
- Infected wounds: Garlic juice with distilled water (1:3), employed as a lotion.

GINGER (*Adrakh*)

Ginger is considered as the universal medicine. A good digestive aid, it thins the blood, lowers blood cholesterol, cleanses the throat and tongue and reduces fever. Also good as a tonic, for colds, cough, asthma and relieves nausea. Good for the lungs, stomach, spleen and neurological diseases. In ancient times, raw ginger was used as a breath sweetener, an aid to digestion, a cure for toothache and bleeding gums and as a strengthening agent for loose teeth and weak eyes.

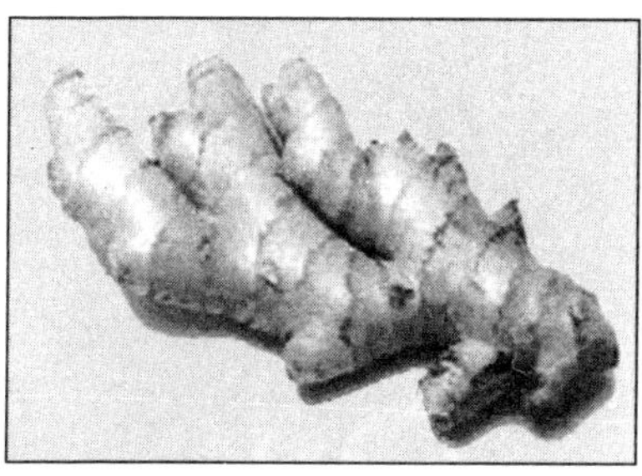

As Medicine:

- Joint pain, rheumatic pain: A paste of dried ginger and asafoetida in milk is applied on the affected area. The area is then exposed to the sun for warmth.
- Dyspepsia, nausea, indigestion, jaundice, morning sickness and piles: Equal quantities of ginger juice, lemon juice, pudina juice and honey, to be taken frequently.
- Indigestion: Grind 1 tsp each saunf, dried ginger and cloves into a fine powder. Add honey to make a thick paste and take 1 tsp after each meal.
- Loss of appetite, stomachache: 1 inch piece of dried ginger is boiled in 2 cups water. After mixing it with milk and sugar, take it frequently like tea.
- Earache: A few drop of ginger juice can be used as

eardrops.

- Toothache and gum inflammation: Apply ginger paste and salt on gums.
- Cold and cough: Prepare a tea of ½ tsp each ginger paste, cloves and cinnamon powder. Add honey and drink. Juice of ginger should be taken with honey 2-3 times daily in persistent cough.
- Boils: Apply a paste of ginger powder and turmeric (1:1) on boils.
- Facial wrinkles and premature graying: Soak shredded ginger in honey. Eat a spoonful every morning.

LEMON (*Nimbu*)

Lemons, one of the most highly alkalinizing foods, are native to tropical Asia. The best lemons have skin of an oily, fine texture and are heavy for their size. Lemon juice makes a good substitute for vinegar. Fresh lemon juice is an outstanding source of vitamin C. Lemons are high in potassium and rich in vitamin B1. They are ideal for getting rid of toxic materials in the body. In many cases, they will help stir up any latent toxic settlements in the body that cannot be eliminated by other ways. Lemon drinks help tremendously when we need to remove the impurities and the fermentative effects of a bad liver.

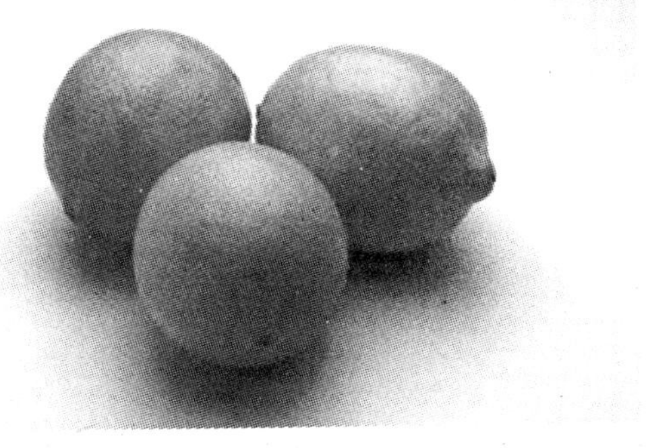

Lemons are wonderful for fevers, because a feverish body responds to citric fruits better than any other food. The lemon seems to have the properties of increasing elimination through the skin and therefore helps reduce the fever. The lemon is a wonderful germicide. There are at least twenty different germs that can be destroyed by the use of the lemon itself. Lemons have been used as a household remedy for colds, rheumatism, sore throat, gastric and liver troubles, headache, heartburn, biliousness etc. Local application of lemon juice is used to allay irritation caused by insect bites.

As Medicine:

- A little lemon and the yolk of a raw egg in a glass of orange juice is an excellent mild laxative, as well as a nutritious drink.
- Drinking of lemon juice daily helps to alleviate rheumatic fever, painful joints, lumbago and sciatica.
- Lemon juice taken three or four times daily along with garlic cures cough and cold.
- Asthma is relieved by taking a half-spoonful of lemon-juice before each meal and upon retiring.
- To avoid travel sickness, a glass of lemon juice should be taken before leaving home.
- Lemon juice rubbed in the scalp before shampooing is an effective remedy for dandruff. Lemon juice also makes a nice rinse for the hair. It removes the soap film much better than plain water.
- Lemon juice is an excellent blood purifier. Upon rising in the morning, drink the juice of one lemon in a cup of warm water. It also helps in reducing obesity.
- If you have ulcers, avoid lemons and other citrus fruits.

MINT (*Pudina*)

The plant belonging to the genus Mentha is an aromatic herb. The chief constituents for which this plant is valued are Menthol and Peppermint oil.

The mint oil is largely used in medicine for stomach disorders, in ointment for headaches, rheumatic and other pains and in cough drops, inhalations, mouthwashes, etc. The oil is also antiseptic.

The dried leaves and flowering tops of the plant constitute the drug Peppermint. The drug is used in treatment of flatulence, vomiting, diarrhoea and nausea. Bruised leaves are applied in headache and other pains.

Mint has many culinary uses and can be used as a flavouring agent in curries or as an appetizer in the form of chutney or jal-jeera drink. As a medicinal herb mint is soothing as well as gently stimulating to the whole of the digestive system, and it is comforting to know that mint is completely safe to use.

As Medicine:

- Powdered dried mint leaves mixed with salt should be used as tooth powder for all kinds of dental problems.
- A mixture of equal quantities of mint leaf juice, lemon juice and honey, taken two tb sp thrice a day before meals is good for any kind of digestive disorder.
- Mint paste in lemon juice applied on the skin gets rid of pimples and blackheads.
- A decoction of boiled mint leaves and green cardamom is good for nausea and indigestion.
- Mint leaf juice applied on the forehead relieves headache and tension.
- Mint leaf juice drops are effective in ear and nose infections.

ONION (*Piyaz*)

Onions, besides having a universal gastronomical appeal, is one of the earliest known food medicines, and was used for hundreds of years for colds and catarrhal disorders and to drive fermentations and impurities out of the system.

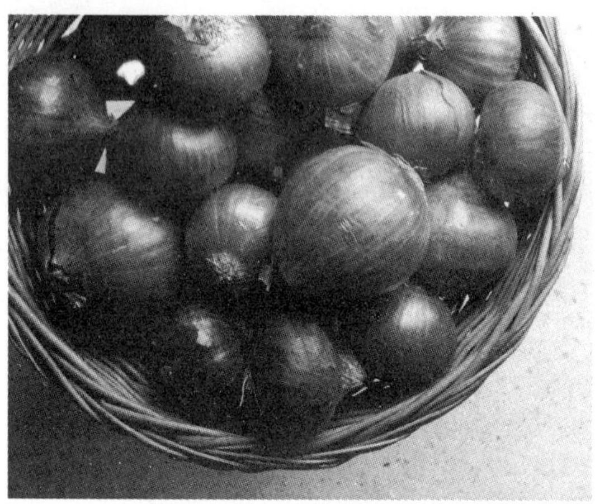

Effective as a poultice, applied to the chest for colds, congestions, and bronchitis and on the ear for ear infections. The onion is described as an antiseptic, stimulant, diuretic and expectorant. If eaten raw at dinnertime, the onion ensures a good night's sleep. For a bad cold and cough there exists nothing better than the consumption of well-boiled or fried onions.

Onions contain a large amount of sulphur and are especially good for the liver.

There is experimental evidence to prove that other than having definite anti-tumour properties, the essential oils found in the onion prevents the deposition of cholesterol in the arteries.

As Medicine:

- Crushed onion or its juice is applied over skin diseases and insect bites; its paste is applied with salt on unbroken chilblains.
- A compress made of a roasted bulb applied on inflamed or protruded piles gives definite relief.
- In malarial fevers, onions are eaten twice a day with 2-3 black peppers with remarkable relief.
- The liquid from a raw onion that has been chopped up fine, covered with honey, and left standing for four to five hours, makes an excellent cough syrup. It is wonderful for soothing an inflamed throat.
- Onion packs on the chest have been used for years in bronchial inflammations.
- Equal quantities of onion juice mixed with warm mustard oil is good as a liniment for arthritis and painful joints
- Equal quantity of raw onion juice and honey, taken twice a day are effective for stomachache and indigestion.
- Raw onion juice as eardrops is effective for ear infections and inflammations.
- Crushed onion paste applied on the head relieves headache.
- A poultice of roasted and crushed onion applied on skin eruptions and boils help them to heal faster.
- For shock and giddiness, fresh crushed onions should be inhaled.

OKRA (*Bhindi*)

The sodium content of okra is very high. It also contains mucin, which protects the internal membranes and soothes the irritated membranes of the intestinal tract. Okra has an alkaline reaction.

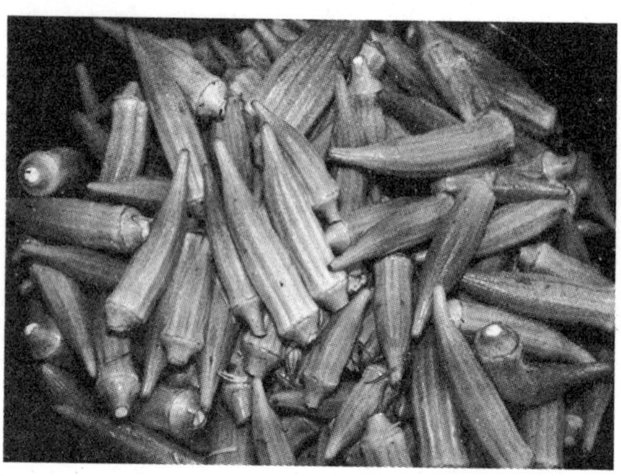

As Medicine:

- Diabetics should eat bhindi regularly as it helps in lowering the blood sugar.
- The water of raw bhindis soaked overnight taken regularly for a month shows remarkable fall in the blood cholesterol and sugar levels.
- Applying raw bhindi paste helps to heal burns and any kind of skin rashes.

PEAS (*Matar*)

Peas contain high amount of fibre, vitamins A, B and C and no fat, making them a good cancer fighter. They also help control blood sugar level and may lower blood pressure.

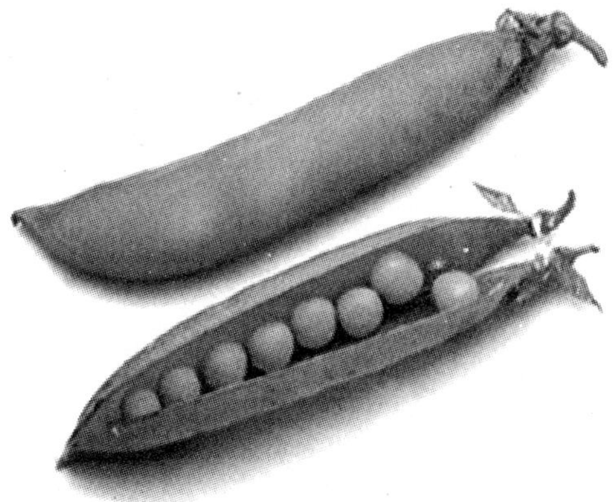

Green peas are very useful in weakness, general debility, anaemia, and in run-down conditions. Hence are known as 'poor man's eggs'.

Fresh garden peas are slightly diuretic in action. They also give relief to ulcer pains because they help use up the stomach acids.

As Medicine:

- Boiled green peas should be taken daily by patients of any blood disorders. The protein of peas has a clot dissolving property.
- Water of boiled dried peas should be used for washing the face to remove the chickenpox marks.
- Tender pea pods are rich in vitamins and minerals and should be cooked as a vegetable for patients of vitamin deficiencies and general weakness.

POTATO (*Aloo*)

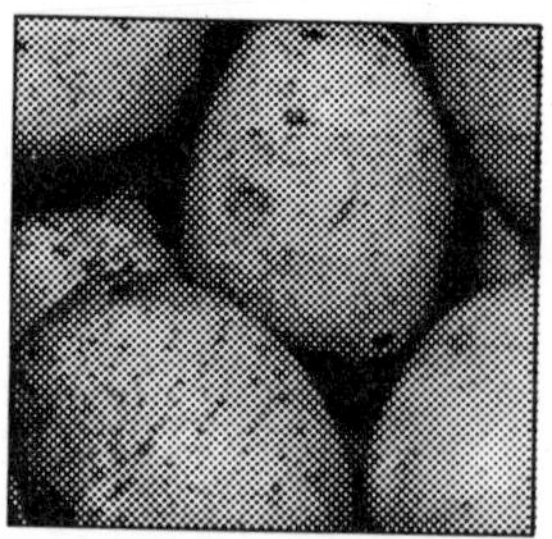

Potato is an almost perfect food, lowering blood pressure, maintaining balance of alkalinity and acidity in the body and rich in vitamins A, B, and C and potassium. (60 percent of the potassium contained in the potato lies so close to the skin that it cannot be saved if the potato is peeled.)

Raw potato juice is a great rejuvenator and is quick way to get an abundance of vitamin C as well as other vitamins and minerals. Potatoes should be avoided if you are suffering from arthritis.

Potato soup is good in cases of uric acid, kidney and stomach disorders, and for replacing minerals in the system. The potassium in the potato is strongly alkaline, which makes for good liver activation and neutralizing acidity.

As Medicine:

- Small potatoes cooked in their jackets as vegetable, if eaten regularly, would diminish all chances of stone formation in the kidneys.
- Potatoes baked in their skin and eaten with salt, reduces fat in the body.
- A cup of raw potato juice taken daily cures acidity.
- Raw potato paste applied on the face, allowed to dry before washing it off, removes wrinkles, clears the skin and makes it glow.
- Raw potato (juice or slices) helps to heal burns faster.
- Boiled potato mashed in milk is an excellent remedy for diarrhoea.
- If eaten daily, potatoes should be cooked in combination with other vegetables, otherwise they might cause constipation.

PUMPKIN (*Kaddu*)

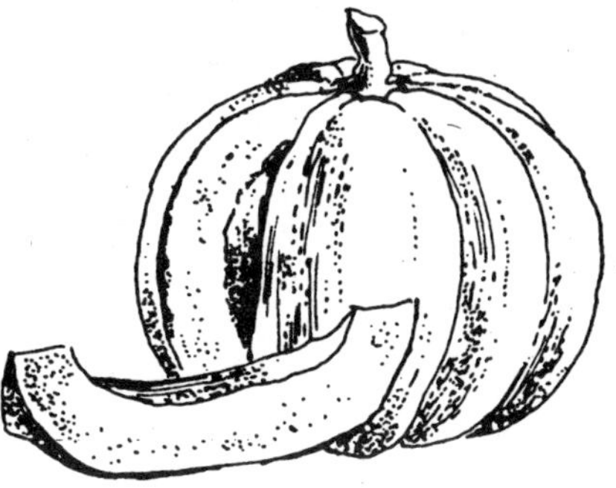

Pumpkins are very high in potassium and sodium. They are alkaline in reaction and are a fair source of vitamins B and C.

Pumpkin juice is very useful in cases of sunstroke, heat stroke, acidity, and liver troubles. It keeps the body cool during hot summer months.

Pumpkin juice is often applied externally on the face to remove dirt, black spots, and to make the skin soft and lovely.

Pumpkin seed is rich in zinc, calcium and B vitamins. The oil and seeds are used to treat the prostate gland. It is used to destroy parasites (worms) in the intestinal tract.

As Medicine:

- Pumpkin seeds and onions mixed together with a little soya milk and honey, taken daily for a week, makes a great remedy for parasitic worms in the digestive tract.
- Juice of fresh ripe pumpkin taken regularly helps to get rid of kidney stones.
- Cooked pumpkin eaten daily in the diet, prevents cancers.
- A poultice of raw pumpkin pulp is good for migraine headaches.

RADISH (*Mooli*)

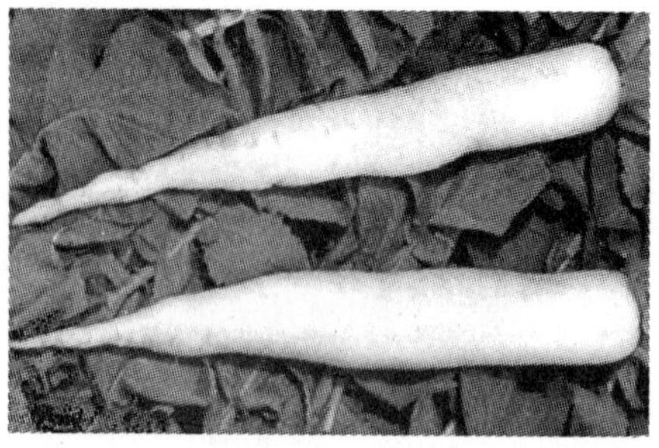

In Chinese medicine the radish is used to promote digestion, remove mucous, soothe headaches and heal laryngitis. The juice is mixed with ginger juice to cure laryngitis.

Radish contains vitamin C in plenty and appreciable amounts of vitamin B complex. The juice of fresh radishes including the leaves is too potent to be taken alone.

Radishes are strongly diuretic and stimulate the appetite and digestion. The juice of raw radishes is helpful in catarrhal conditions. The mustard oil content of the radish makes it good for expelling gallstones from the bladder.

As Medicine:

- Raw radish taken daily as salad, helps in maintaining the health of kidneys, and also helps in the digestion of starchy foods.
- Juice of radish and its leaves, mixed with a little sugar, should be taken twice daily in the cases of jaundice.
- A poultice of raw crushed radish is effective for insect bites and stings.
- Equal quantities of radish juice, cucumber juice and capsicum juice, taken once a week would help in cleansing the digestive and respiratory systems of the body.

SPINACH (*Palak*)

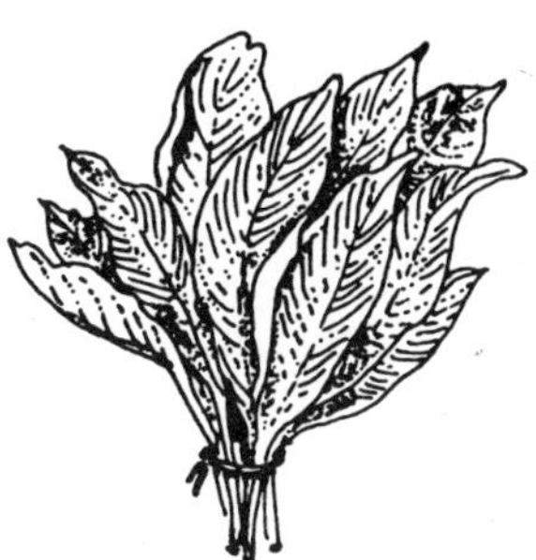

Spinach has been both praised and abused. It is praised because of its health benefits and abused for its smell and flavour (which can be looked after by the cooks). To retain its best qualities, spinach should be steamed or cooked in minimum water.

Spinach is an excellent source of vitamins C and A, and iron and potassium. Spinach has a laxative effect and is wonderful in weight-loss diets.

The leaves are valuable in cases of pernicious anaemia, low vitality and neuralgia.

Spinach is good for those who are in need of iron, taking spinach leaf juice either raw or by cooking as stew or soups.

This juice is rich in all minerals and organic substances and is good as a cleansing blood tonic, healing the intestinal tract, haemorrhoids, anaemia and vitamin deficiencies.

Spinach has high calcium content, but also contains oxalic acid. The oxalic acid prohibits the absorption of calcium by the body. For this reason, those who have known liver disease, kidney stones or arthritis should eat spinach sparingly.

As Medicine:

- Cooked spinach vegetable, taken regularly, protects against cancer.
- Raw spinach juice taken twice a day before meals lowers the blood sugar.
- Spinach leaf juice, as a gargle, is good for sore throat.

TOMATO (*Tamatar*)

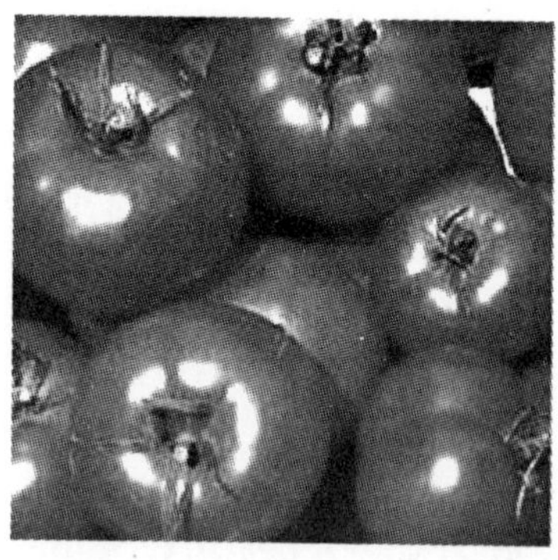

Contrary to popular belief, tomato is not acid forming; it contains a great deal of citric acid but is alkaline when it enters the blood stream. It increases the alkalinity of the blood and helps remove toxins, especially uric acid, from the system. As a liver cleanser, tomatoes are wonderful, especially when used with the green vegetable juices.

Tomatoes are the richest of all foods in vitamins. They are very rich in the important vitamins like A, B and C. Unripe or half-ripe tomatoes are also effective in stomach disorders.

It is easily digestible and is recommended for invalids and especially in fevers, diabetes and after long fasts. Being a rich source of vitamin A, it is a dependable preventive against eye troubles. It contains other minerals like iron, calcium, sulphur and potassium also.

As Medicine:

- A glass of fresh tomato juice taken daily cleanses the system and prevents hardening of the arteries.
- Tomato juice keeps the blood stream alkaline and thus maintains high resistance to disease.
- Being a rich source of vitamin A, it is a dependable preventive against eye troubles.
- Half-ripe tomatoes are very useful in hot summer months as they prevent sunstroke or heat stroke.

TURNIP (*Shalgam*)

Turnips are very rich in vitamins A, B and C. They are very useful in cases of rapid pulse, physical weakness, tender joints, stammering, catarrh, poor appetite and digestive disturbances.

Turnip leaves contain more calcium than any other vegetable. Cooked as any other leafy green vegetable, it is an excellent food for growing children.

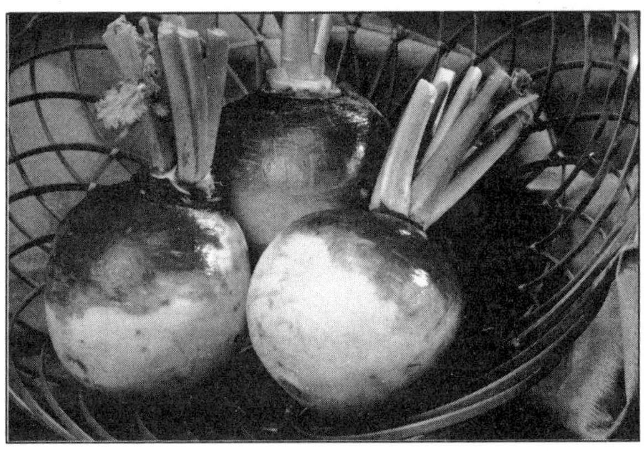

Turnip juice has twice the amount of vitamin C as oranges or tomatoes. Turnips are also good for the elimination of uric acid from the body, which is good for the overweight persons and gout sufferers. Turnips are very high in sulphur and are sometimes gas forming. When fresh and young, turnips can be used raw in salads.

As Medicine:

- Turnip juice is especially good for any mucous and catarrhal conditions.
- Turnip juice mixed with cabbage or carrot juice, taken daily reduces mucous, helps asthma and bronchitis and relieves sore throats.

- Turnip packs over the chest are good for relieving bronchial disorders and packs over the throat are good for sore throats.
- Turnip leaves are considered good for controlling calcium in the body, as are all other greens. They have been used successfully to combat diseases caused by lack of calcium in the body.
- If you have arthritis and need to omit oranges and tomatoes from your diet, use turnips to provide yourself with a source rich in the vitamin C you need.
- Turnips are good for the elimination of uric acid and kidney stones derived from uric acid.
- Boiled turnip taken once a week reduces the blood cholesterol.
- To cure constipation, steamed turnip with lemon juice and salt should be eaten daily.

MUSHROOMS

Mushroom is a kind of fungus. Mushrooms have been credited with various curative properties like removing warts and blemishes on the skin, curing madness and now scientists are trying to identify anti-cancer properties in them.

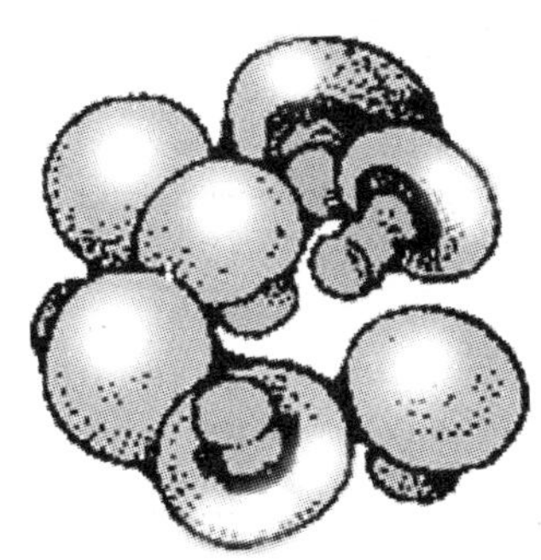

There are more than 13000 varieties of edible mushrooms. Mushrooms have a distinct flavour. Most edible varieties have a special odour and very pleasant taste. There are many varieties of mushrooms in India, but all are not safe to eat. A number of them are, in fact poisonous. Unfortunately, there is no easy way of recognizing a poisonous variety. Therefore, it is advisable to eat only cultivated ones.

The food value of mushrooms is somewhere between that of vegetables and animal foods. Most mushrooms are a fair source of proteins and contain low amounts of starch. Some of them are rich in B complex vitamins and minerals like iron and copper. Certain kinds of anaemias are reported to have been treated successfully with mushroom extracts. Most of the vitamins in the mushrooms are retained even when cooked, canned, dehydrated or frozen.

FRUITS

No other class of edible plants has such variety of pleasant and attractive flavours. The nutritive value of fruits is much less important. The only essential nutrient in which fruits are rich is ascorbic acid or vitamin C. Almost all fruits contain significant amount of this vitamin and some are quite rich in it.

Fruits, like vegetables, also contain fibre, making them good natural laxatives. That is why; people with sensitive stomachs can take fruit only in small amounts. Most fruits contain small quantities of carotene and the B group of vitamins. The amounts present are not usually great but may help, like for instance, there is always an improvement in the children's health during the season of mangoes, when they consume huge quantities of the fruit. (Mangoes have carotene, which gets converted into vitamin A in the body.)

Fruits contain little or no protein or fat. Most contain 5 – 20% of carbohydrates. Ripe fruits contain no starch. Fructose and glucose are the chief sugars found.

Fruits contain organic acids, which are responsible for the sourness of unripe fruits. During ripening, the concentration of these acids falls and that of sugars rises. In any case the body easily oxidizes these acids and excretes them. Fruits do not cause acidosis.

Fruits should be eaten seasonally and ripe fruit is best to eat. Unlike vegetables, fruits are eaten uncooked, so there are very few medicinal recipes available. Also, in most of the cases the bark of the fruit tree, its leaves or its seeds are used in traditional medicine more than the commonly available fruit.

APPLE (*Seb*)

Apples are an alkaline food. They are also an eliminative food, and contain pectin, which has the ability to take up excess water in the intestines and make a soft bulk that acts as a mild, non-irritating stimulant. This stimulant helps the peristaltic movement and aids in natural bowel elimination.

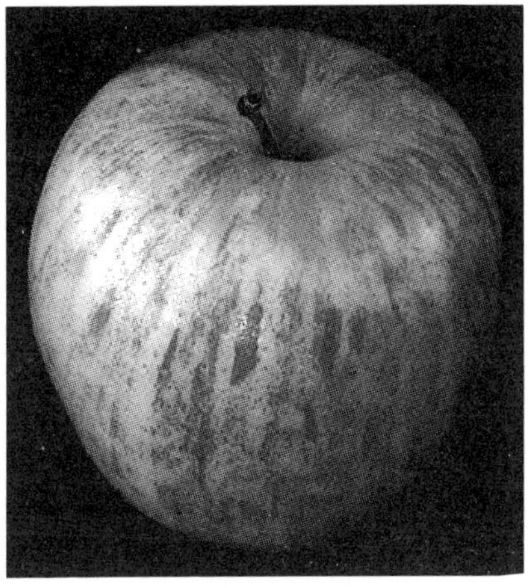

Though the iron content of the apple is not high, it has a property that helps the body absorb the iron from other foods.

Apples contain 50 percent more vitamin A than oranges. This vitamin helps ward off colds and other infections and promotes growth.

It also keeps the eyes in good condition, and prevents night blindness.

Apples are rich in vitamin C, which is a body normalizer and is essential in keeping bones and teeth sound. The vitamin that is so important in maintaining nerve health, vitamin B is also found in apples.

Apple juice is good for the gall bladder and is known for its cleansing and healing effects on internal inflammation. Apples can lower blood cholesterol, aid liver function, rid the body of toxins and lessen the effects of X-rays.

The fruit is best taken raw or cooked (steamed).

As Medicine:

- Apples are considered valuable as anti-scorbutic fruits. Regular intake of apples ensures overall health, especially that of skin, bones and teeth.
- Steamed apples, being rich in pectin, are useful in diarrhoea.
- Apple murabba acts as a heart stimulant and is also reported to relieve mental strain.

APRICOT (*Khubani*)

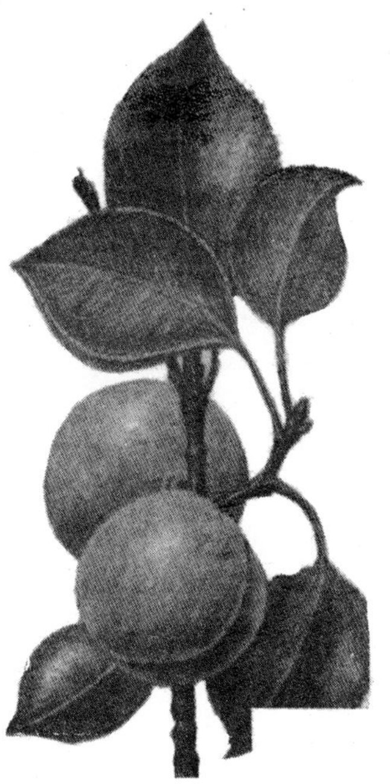

The seeds are used in cancer treatment. They contain a chemical, which is believed to be beneficial in controlling cancer. Apricots contain good amounts of potassium, iron and are good sources of vitamin A and are high in natural sugar content. Dried apricots are an excellent source of iron. Apricots also contain cobalt, which is necessary in the treatment of anaemic conditions.

Dried apricots have six times as much sugar content as the fresh fruit.

Therefore, persons with diabetes must be careful not to eat too much dried apricots. However, they are good when an energy boost is needed.

The fruit is best taken raw or cooked (steamed).

As Medicine:

- Apricot kernel oil is used for earache.
- Steamed apricots are advised to persons suffering from fever as they have a cooling effect.
- Apricots are also useful as a laxative.

AMLA (*Gooseberry*)

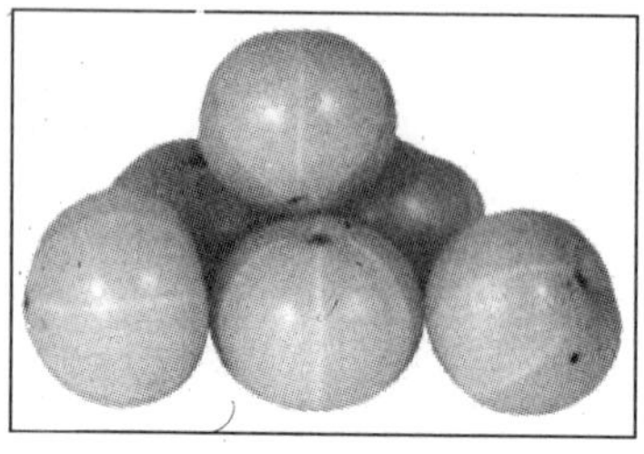

The ripe fruits are yellowish-green, fleshy and are very rich in vitamin C. Fruits are pickled and also eaten fresh.

Amla fruit has been held in high esteem in indigenous medicine. It is acidic, cooling, refrigerant, diuretic and laxative. In combination with iron, amla is used as a remedy for anaemia, jaundice and dyspepsia. Amla is one of the three ingredients in Triphala, a compound in indigenous medicine, used in the treatment of headache, biliousness, dyspepsia, constipation, enlarged liver and ascites.

As Medicine:

- Constipation: Soak 1 or 2 dried fruits in water overnight. Mash and filter the next morning. Add 1 tsp honey and drink.
- Urinary problems: Soak separately 2 tsp each dried amla and raisins in water overnight. Mash, filter and drink the next morning. Continue for a few days.
- Headache, heaviness in head: Grind the fresh fruits into a fine paste and apply on affected parts.
- Skin-problem: Grind the dried fruits into a fine powder and use as a substitute for soap.
- Anxiety, loss of appetite: Remove seeds from fresh fruits and grind the pulp into a fine paste. Take it in a muslin cloth and squeeze out the juice. Take 2 tsp of this juice and mix it with two spoonfuls each honey and limejuice. Add one teacup water and drink on an empty stomach every morning.

BEL (*Wood Apple*)

The bel fruit is very useful in treating chronic diarrhoea and dysentery, particularly for patients having diarrhoea alternating with spells of constipation. Sharbat prepared from the pulp of the fruits is useful as a soothing agent for the intestines of patients who have just recovered from bacillary dysentery. The unripe or half-ripe fruits improve appetite and digestion.

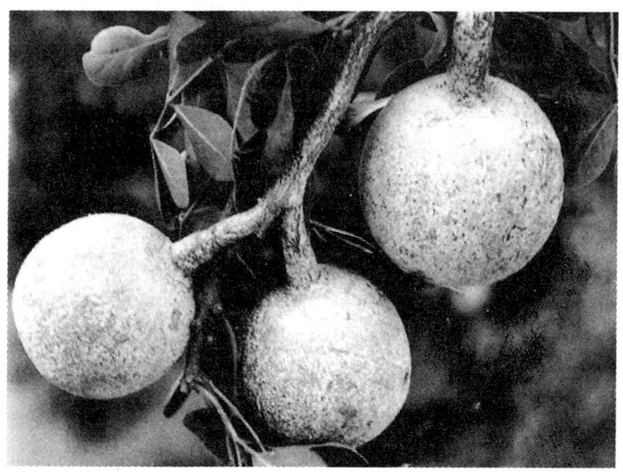

As Medicine:

- Constipation, dyspepsia and mouth ulcers: Mix the pulp of a fruit with jaggery and eat once a day.
- Dysentery: Take 1 teacup fruit pulp twice a day.
- Ulcer in stomach: Mix 1 teacup pulp with 1 tsp sugar and eat early morning on an empty stomach for 3 days.
- Piles, haemorrhoids: Take an unripe fruit and pound it along with 1 tsp each dried ginger and saunf and soak these in 4 teacups of water and sip this water 3 to 4 times a day.

BANANA (*Kela*)

Banana contains many vitamins and minerals, and a great deal of fibre. The ripe fruit is a mild laxative. The unripe fruit is very good for all sorts of stomach and liver troubles, including gastric ulcer. Banana feeds the natural acidophilus bacteria of the bowel, and its high potassium content benefits the muscular system. Its energy content makes it a very advantageous and filling staple, though poorer in proteins as compared to cereals. The banana is a fair source of B vitamins, calcium and phosphorus.

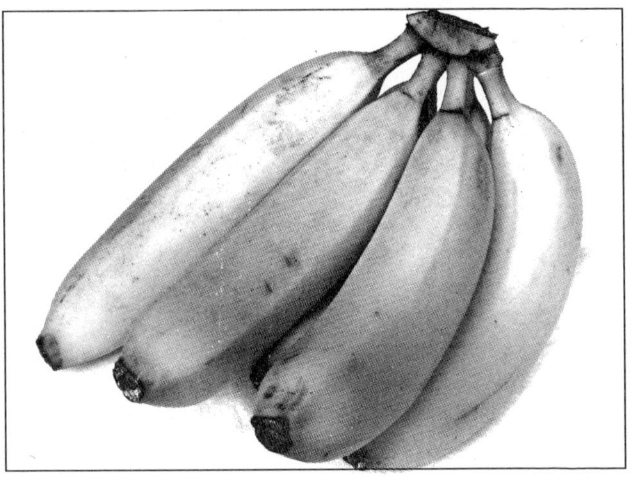

Ripe bananas can augment the diets of small children and convalescents with much beneficial effect. They are very easily digested and the nutrients are absorbed well. Mashed banana with milk and sugar is an excellent supplementary or weaning food for children. Because of their high energy content, bananas are also used in the diets of children being treated for severe malnutrition. An interesting thing about banana is that it is good both for constipation as well as diarrhoea and dysentery.

As Medicine:

- An ounce of the ripe fruit mixed with tamarind and salt is an excellent remedy in early cases of diarrhoea and dysentery.
- Constipation, general weakness and intestinal ulcers: Regular intake of ripe banana.
- Indigestion: Take a ripe banana along with a cup of milk at bedtime.
- Piles: Boil a mashed ripe banana in 1 teacup milk and take twice or thrice a day.
- Cough: Mix $^1/_4$ tsp black pepper powder with a mashed ripe banana and eat twice or thrice a day.
- TB: Mash a ripe banana along with $^1/_2$ cup curd, 1 tsp honey and 1 teacup coconut water and take twice a day.
- Jaundice and typhoid: Mash a ripe banana along with 1 tbsp honey and eat twice a day for a few days.

DATE (*Khajoor*)

The natural sugar contained in the date is much better than highly refined white sugar.

The fruit is very good for cough and cold, asthma, laryngitis, chest complaints, fevers, dysentery and liver complaints. Taking dates with milk early in the morning during winter months is found to be a good tonic. Dates can be eaten with milk for ulcers of the stomach. The date water can be used with milk for children who have sensitive stomachs, as it helps digest the milk.

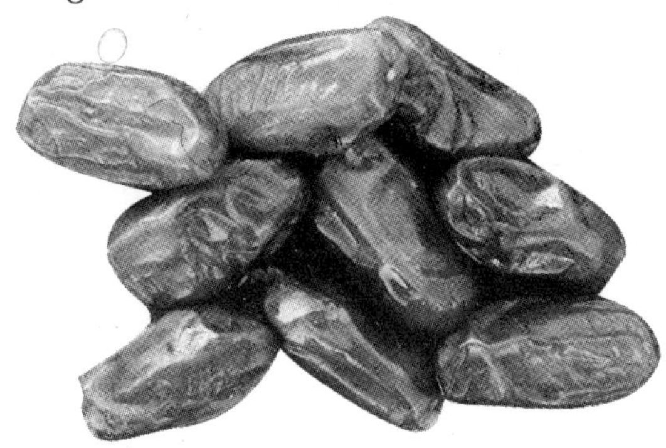

The fibre of cellulose of the date is very soft and does not irritate the stomach. Dates are heat producing, and give energy to people who engage in physical exercise and hard work. They are also a good source of copper, which is a diet essential, even though it is needed by the body only in small amounts.

As Medicine:

- Dates are demulcent, expectorant and laxative and are used in respiratory and digestive disorders.
- Dates are also reported to be effective in cases of memory disturbance.
- Dried dates soaked in milk are highly nutritious and give energy and vitality.

FIG (*Anjir*)

Fig juice is good for destroying intestinal parasites. It has a definite laxative effect and a high alkalinity. The laxative effect is due to the bulk of seeds and fibre combined with mucin and pectin present in the juice. A decoction of dried figs is an excellent mouthwash for sore throat and aphthous complaints of the mouth.

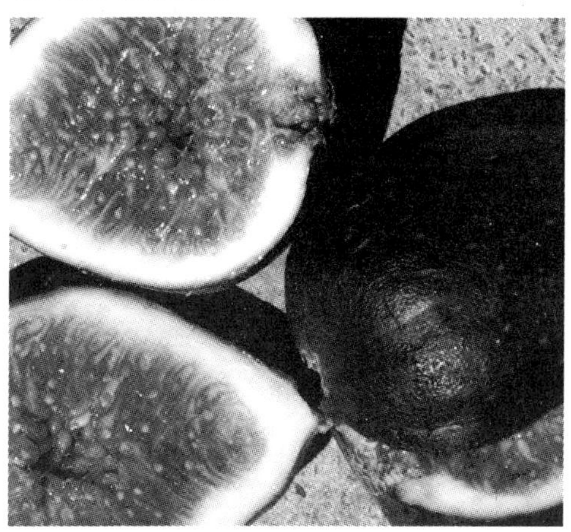

They are best eaten raw and fresh. They are a high calcium food, high in carbohydrates, which gets converted into energy very quickly. They are also known to have some anti-cancer properties.

As Medicine:

- Anaemia: Soak 2 or 3 dried figs overnight in 1 teacup water. Eat them along with milk the next morning, and continue for a month.
- Diabetes: Eat 1 tsp seeds of the fig, separated from the pulp, along with 1 tsp honey every day for a few weeks.
- Inflammation of spleen: Eat 2 or 3 figs along with 1 teacup curd twice a day for a few weeks.
- Constipation: Take 2 or 3 figs after each meal.

- Kidney and/or bladder stones: Consume 1 teacup juice of fresh figs frequently. Boil 2 small fig pieces in 1 teacup water. Take 2 to 3 times daily for a few weeks.
- Boils, small tumours: Roast a fresh fig and cut into half. Make a poultice and apply.
- Early stages of Chickenpox: Include figs in your diet every day.
- Dry cough, liver problem and physical weakness: Soak 2 or 3 dried figs overnight in 1 teacup water. Eat them along with 1 tbsp honey the next morning. Continue for a month.

GRAPEFRUIT (*Chakotra*)

Grapefruit is rich in vitamins C and B. It is low in calories, which makes it good for a weight reducing diet. There is less sugar in grapefruit than in oranges.

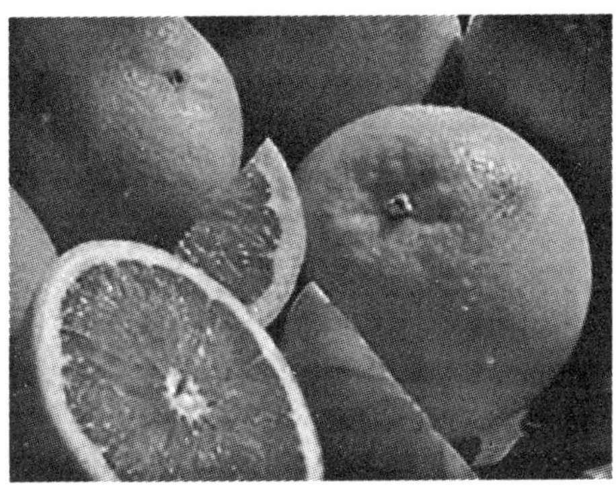

Grapefruit is very rich in citric acid, potassium and calcium, making it good for general weakness. When taken at bedtime, grapefruit is conducive to a sound sleep. A drink of grapefruit juice first thing in the morning helps prevent constipation. It is also an excellent aid in reducing fevers from colds and flu, and seldom causes allergic reactions. The sour taste of grapefruit increases the flow of digestive juices in the stomach. Grapefruit served at the beginning of a meal stimulates the appetite and helps in digestion.

As Medicine:

- For constipation, drink half a glass of grapefruit juice with a pinch of salt, first thing in the morning, on an empty stomach.
- For sleeplessness, take a glass of grapefruit juice with a teaspoonful of sugar, at bedtime.
- For loss of appetite and taste, take half a glass of grapefruit juice with a pinch of black salt, before meals.

GUAVA (*Amrud*)

Fresh guavas are rich in vitamins A, B and C. Guava, other than being a naturally excellent source of vitamin C (it is the richest source of vitamin C after Amla), is also a good laxative. The high fibre content of guava helps in the control of blood sugar and cholesterol levels, apart from relieving cough and related chest problems. Because of its high vitamin C content, it is also good for bleeding gums and joint pains. It also gives the skin a healthy glow. It increases the body's resistance to disease. (This is perhaps nature's way of helping us to combat coughs and colds in this weather!)

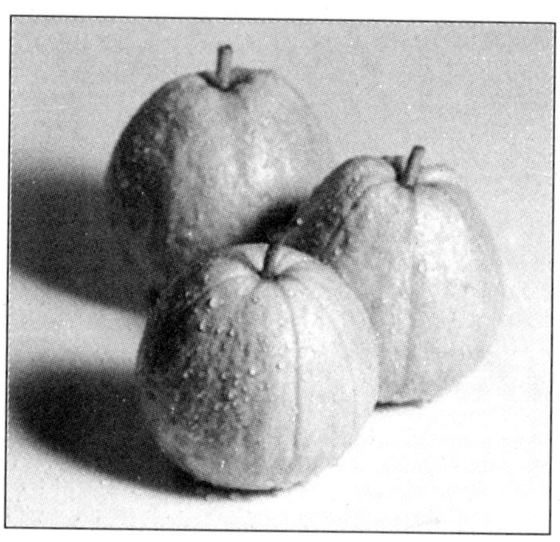

As Medicine:

- The fruit is astringent in action and is good (after scooping out the seeds) for diarrhoea and dysentery.
- Fully ripe fruit, regularly taken cooked as a vegetable, gets rid of obstinate constipation.
- Regular intake of guava ensures the building up of body's resistance against cough and cold; and also makes the skin glow.

LIME (*Mosambi*)

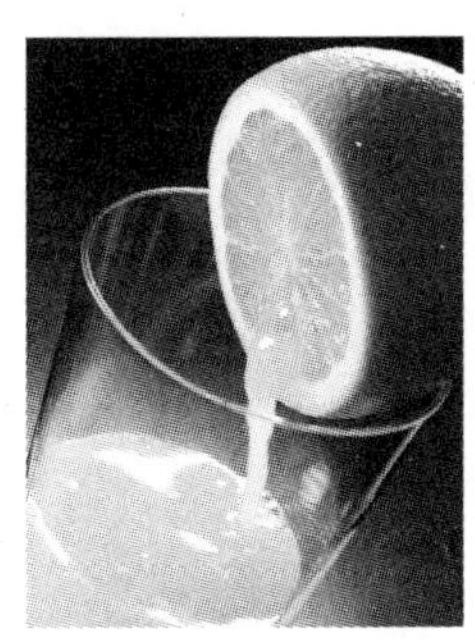

Lime contains vitamins A, B and C. It also contains various other minerals and acids. The fruit juice is an efficacious remedy in scurvy, anaemia, intestinal disorders, cough and cold, gastric troubles, constipation, fevers, typhoid and high blood pressure.

Limes are good in arthritis because they have a high vitamin C content, which dissolves the salts that form in the arthritic joints. They are especially good for anyone with acidity, because they are one of the most alkalinizing foods. A drink of limejuice and whey is a wonderful coolant for the brain and nervous system. Limes can be used to treat brain fever, or someone who is mentally ill. Limes make a wonderful sedative.

As Medicine:

- Swelling and pain in legs/hands: Mix equal quantities of castor oil and limejuice. Massage the affected area with this mixture.
- Diabetes: Mix 2 tsp limejuice in 4 tsp amla juice and 1 tsp honey. Take every morning on an empty stomach.
- To prevent constipation: Take limejuice mixed with warm water at daybreak.
- Feverishness, nausea etc: Mix equal quantities of fresh limejuice in tender coconut water and drink.
- Bad breath, mouth ulcers: Drink lime juice in warm water after frequent gargling. Repeat.
- Black spots, blemishes, pimples: Apply fresh limejuice on the affected areas before going to bed. Wash them with warm water next morning.
- Dehydration: Add salt and sugar to lime juice, mix well and drink.
- Dizziness, stomach distress, nausea, indigestion: Frequent intake of lime juice is recommended.

MANGO (*Aam*)

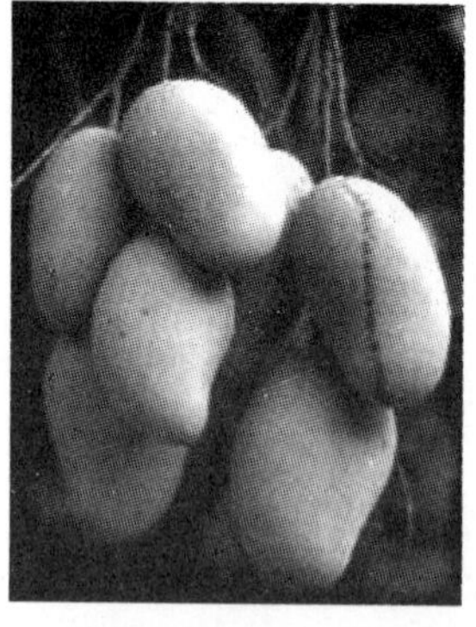

The unripe fruit is acidic and astringent. The ripe fruit is antiscorbutic, diuretic, laxative, invigorating, fattening, and astringent. Sun dried slices of the unripe fruit are very useful in scurvy.

The smoke of the burning leaves is supposed to cure hiccups and some throat troubles and the kernel is effective against diarrhoea and asthma. Baked and sugared pulp is given to patients of cholera and plague. The bark is a source of resins and gum. The gum and the resinous substance exuded by the stem-end of the harvested fruit are mixed with limejuice and given in cases of scabies and cutaneous afflictions.

Few fruits contain as much vitamin A as the mangoes, in addition to having a high content of vitamin C.

As Medicine:

- Spleen enlargement: Add 1 tsp honey to a teacup of ripe mango pulp. Take thrice a day.
- Indigestion and liver trouble: Suck a ripe mango and top it with a glass of milk.
- Baldness: Rub on the scalp 1 tbsp oil in which raw mangoes have been preserved for over one year.
- General weakness: Sprinkle the following on a platter of mango slices: 1 tsp honey, a pinch of saffron, cardamom and rose water. Take twice daily.
- Heat exhaustion, heat stroke: Cook an unripe fruit in hot ashes. Extract the pulp and mix with water and 1 tbsp sugar, and take.
- Prickly heat: Boil 2 raw mangoes in 2 teacups water. Cool. Squeeze out the pulp. Add salt or sugar or both to taste. Drink at least once a day.

MELONS (*Tarbuz*)

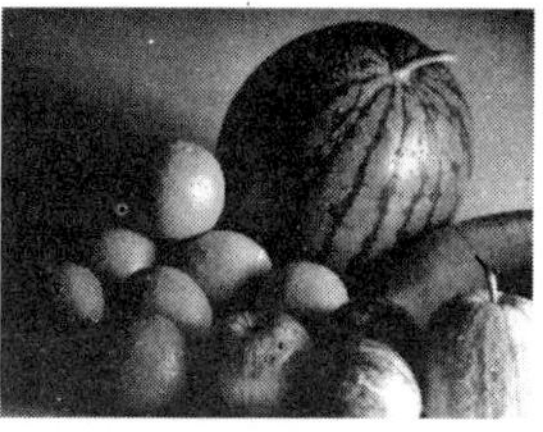

Watermelon (tarbuz) is a large fruit, achieving a diameter of 20 inches at times. The dark-green rind covers a soft, spongy and fleshy inner portion. The pulp is usually reddish-pink with black seeds embedded in it. The watermelon is best consumed in the form of squashes, juice or just as slices. Being a fair source of sodium and potassium it helps to relieve muscular fatigue. The inner portion of the watermelon seeds can be eaten roasted or fried. These seeds contain 34% protein and 52% oil.

Muskmelon (kharbooja) is eaten as a delicacy, because of its typical musk like flavour and taste. It makes a very good ingredient of fruit salads, ice cream and milk shakes.

Muskmelon seeds are also edible, and are used as substitutes for almonds and pistachios in the confectionary industry. The inner portion of the seed is eaten. It is very tasty and is rich in protein (36%) and oil (45%).

Nutritionally speaking, more than 90% of the melon is water. The energy content is 15-25 per cent. However, the deep orange or yellow varieties of muskmelon contain some vitamin A, vitamin C and calcium.

Melons give an excellent supply of distilled water that contains the finest mineral elements possible. Melons, with their root system, pick up water from deep, in-ground reserves, and bring it to our tables in a delicious fruit substance. Melons are excellent for rejuvenation, aiding elimination and alkalinizing the body.

As Medicine:

- They are wonderful diuretic agents. They are of great value in disease of the heart, kidneys and diabetes.
- Because of their high water content, they have a high satiety value and hence are useful in weight reduction diets.

ORANGE (*Santara*)

Oranges contain high amounts of vitamins C and A. Sweet orange juice acts as a mild laxative and is very effective during cough and cold, fevers, general debility, dimness of vision, anaemia, lassitude, constipation, scurvy, and headache. It cures vomiting and checks carsickness. It is very useful in low blood pressure.

It is an excellent food for children as a supplement for those who must drink milk because it seems to help in the retention of calcium in the body. Ripe oranges contain as much as ten percent fruit sugar, which can be immediately assimilated by the body.

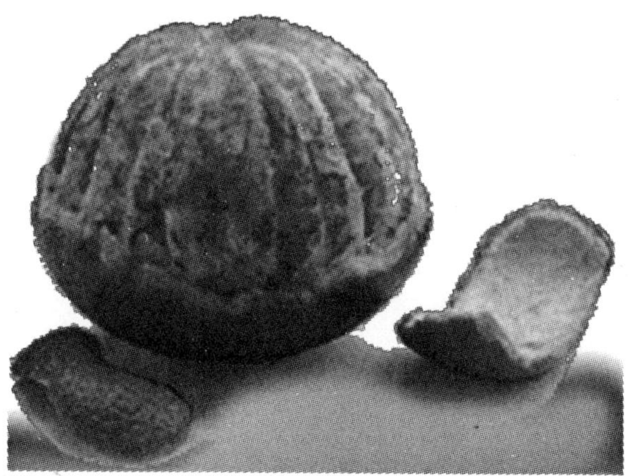

As Medicine:

- Fever: Orange is an excellent food in all types of fever when the digestive power of the body is seriously disturbed. Orange juice is the most ideal liquid food in fevers like typhoid, T.B. and measles. It gives energy, increases urinary output and promotes body resistance against infections, thereby helping to recover fast.

- Dyspepsia: Orange is a good remedy for chronic dyspepsia. It stimulates the flow of digestive juices thereby improving digestion and increasing appetite. It also creates suitable conditions for the development of friendly bacteria in the intestines.
- Bones and Teeth: As it is a good source of Vitamin C, it works well in the diseases of the bones and teeth. Giving large amounts of orange juice can cure pyorrhoea and dental caries. Regular intake of oranges also helps in prevention of arthritis.
- Heart Disease: Orange juice sweetened with honey, is highly useful in heart diseases.
- Acne: The orange peel is valuable in the treatment of pimples and acne. The peel, pounded well with water, should be applied on the affected areas.

PAPAYA (*Papita*)

The chymopapain contained in papaya softens tight muscles and is the reason it is the main ingredient in meat tenderizers. The fruit contains vitamins A, B and C. It is a tonic, laxative, digestive, and rejuvenative. Ripe fruit is very useful in digestive disorders and if taken regularly, it cures all sorts of stomach troubles. The unripe fruit is also prescribed in stomach troubles, jaundice, gastritis and liver disorder. The ripe fruit should be eaten regularly for habitual constipation and chronic diarrhoea.

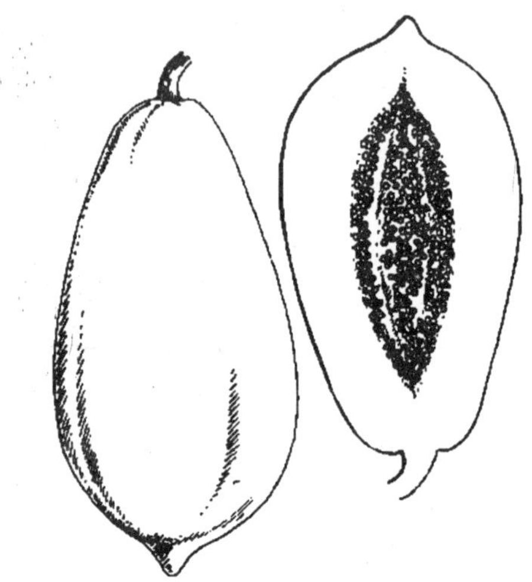

As Medicine:

- The juice is applied on corns, warts, pimples, horny excretions of the skin and other skin diseases.
- Anaemia, constipation, eye-diseases and intestinal worms: Eat papayas frequently.
- Liver and spleen inflammation: Take papaya daily with 1 tsp of honey.
- Dead, flaky skin on face: Take a ripe papaya slice and mash the pulp. Use it as a face pack overnight.

PINEAPPLE (*Ananas*)

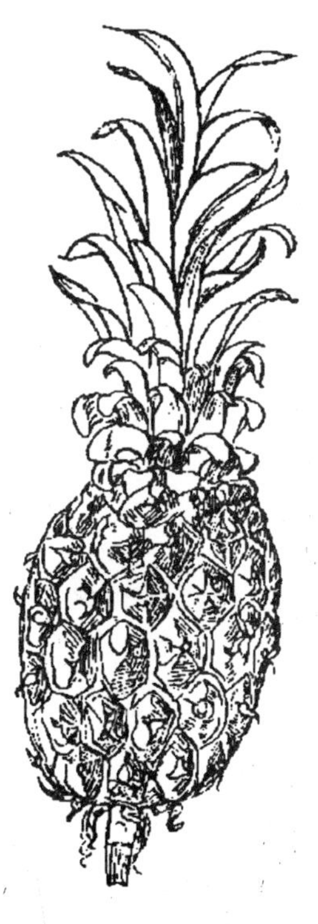

The fruit contains vitamin C, iron and other minerals. It acts as an effective laxative. It is good for constipation and poor digestion. The pineapple helps to digest proteins.

It is a tonic and rejuvenative. Juice of the unripe fruit causes uterine contractions and should not be given to a pregnant woman. Juice of the ripe fruit cures gastric irritability in fever and is very helpful in jaundice.

High in vitamin C the pineapple is considered to be a protective fruit.

As Medicine:

- Fresh pineapple juice contains an enzyme, which aids in digestion.
- The fruit is also antihelminthic in nature, that is, it helps in getting rid of intestinal worms.
- Juice from unripe fruits acts as a strong purgative, useful in constipation.
- Pineapple pieces eaten fresh with salt and pepper help to get rid of indigestion.
- To get rid of kidney stones, pineapple juice should be taken every morning for a month.

POMEGRANATE (*Anar*)

Nutritionally, pomegranate is rich in energy only, providing 90 calories per 100 gm. It is also rich in tannin, which acts as an astringent in the intestines and precipitates food proteins. It is advised in diarrhoea, though there is no evidence of its efficiency in improving this condition.

The juice is one of the best for bladder disorders and has a slight purgative effect. For elderly people it is a wonderful kidney and bladder tonic.

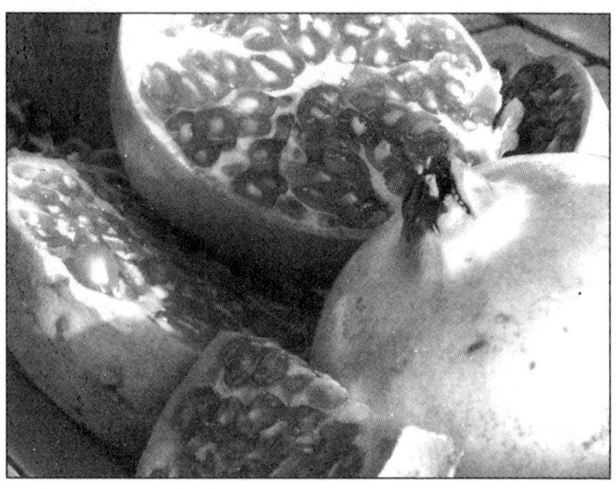

As Medicine:

- Ripe fruit juice is good in typhoid fever, gastric and asthmatic fevers.
- The fruit juice is highly effective in reducing high blood pressure.
- The fruit juice with honey is an age-old remedy for loss of memory.
- Anaemia: Dissolve $^{1}/_{4}$ tsp cinnamon and 2 tsp honey in 1 cup pomegranate juice and drink.
- Asthma, cough: Mix juice of fresh ginger, pomegranate and honey in equal quantities. Take 1 tbsp of this mixture once or twice a day.

PEACH (*Arhoo*)

The peach has a high sugar and water content and hence has a very good laxative effect. Peaches are wonderful in alkalinizing the blood stream and stimulate the digestive juices. They can be used to regulate the bowel and build the blood. Peaches are an excellent food for elderly people, because the body assimilates this food very easily. Because they are easy to digest, very ripe peaches can be eaten in cases of ulcers of the stomach or inflammation of the bowel, and also in cases of colitis. Peaches are wonderful in helping to eliminate toxins from the body, and they are good to eat on a weight-loss programme.

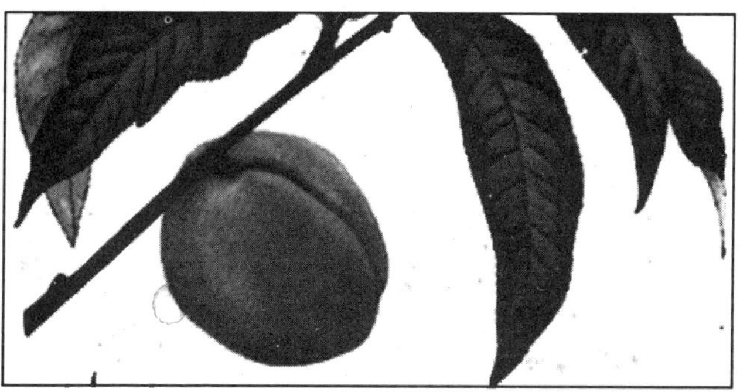

As Medicine:

- Ripe fruits are given in stomach ailments, as they soothe the walls of the stomach and remove all the accumulated toxins from the digestive system.
- Its juice is known to remove worms from the intestine.
- It is also very useful in keeping the eyes healthy.

SPICES

Spices and condiments have always had a special magic about them. They were once a royal luxury and very few except the rich could afford them.

All spices are of plant origin. They can be flowers–cloves, fruits–chillies, seeds–coriander, roots–ginger, leaves–curry leaf, bark–cinnamon, and so on.

Spices and condiments are basically adjuncts that impart a flavour and taste to the foods to which they are added. They not only improve palatability but also perform a very important task of preserving foods for long periods. This is made possible because of the anti-bacterial properties of spices.

It is a very well known fact that salivary and gastric secretions are stimulated by aroma, so it follows that spices aid in digestion by adding a flavour and a tang to the food we eat. Most herbs and spices contain the B complex vitamins, and minerals like iron and calcium in appreciable concentrations. But the quantities eaten are too small to be significant. The energy value and protein content of the spices is negligible, but when these are added, food becomes tastier and people tend to eat more, thus they may take in more nutrients. Some spices such as green chillies are rich in vitamin C, and in poor families they may contribute significantly to the vitamin C content of the diet. 30gm of green chillies would suffice for the whole day's requirement of vitamin C for an adult.

Spices in general are carminative in nature. In constipated persons spices help evacuation of the bowel by irritating the intestines. The Indigenous system of medicine has given an extra special place to spices because of their unique medicinal properties. Clove oil is applied to relieve toothaches. Pepper added to hot tea is a patent 'grandma's treatment' for common cold. Turmeric (haldi) has anti-bacterial properties and its solution can be used as an antiseptic for cleaning wounds.

With all these properties spices also have certain drawbacks associated with them. Too much spice may result in diarrhoea in some people and acidity leading to vomiting in others.

ASAFOETIDA (*Hing*)

It is a very useful remedy for relieving spasms and indigestion, flatulent colic, cholera and whooping cough. It is a stimulant for respiratory and nervous systems and is very effective in pneumonia and bronchitis in children. It is applied externally on the stomach to stimulate the intestines, even its enema is recommended in intestinal fluctuations. Hing is also known to have some sedative properties and its possible use in heart diseases has been suggested.

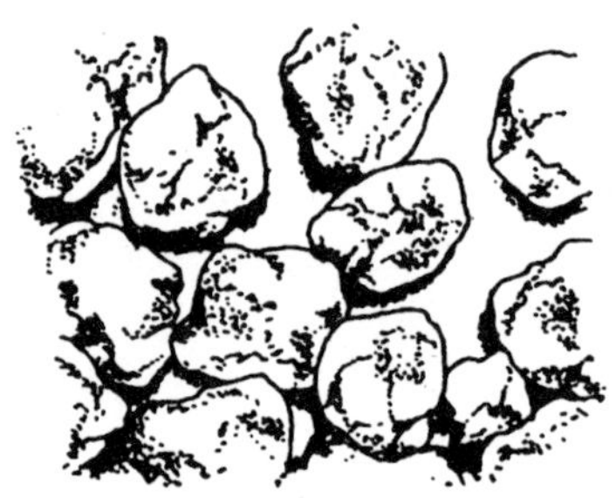

As Medicine:

- Diabetes: Mix $^1/_4$ tsp hing powder in 2 tsp bitter gourd juice. Take twice a day.
- Indigestion: Mix $^1/_4$ tsp hing powder with a ripe banana and eat.
- Stomachache: Dissolve 1 tsp hing in 1 teacup hot water. Drench a cloth pad and foment the abdominal region.
- Kidney-problems: Mix $^1/_4$ tsp hing in 2 tsp fresh ginger juice. Add a pinch of salt and sip.
- Toothache: Heat $^1/_2$ tsp in 2 tsp lemon juice. Soak a piece of cotton in this solution and place it in the tooth cavity.

BISHOP'S WEED (*Ajwain*)

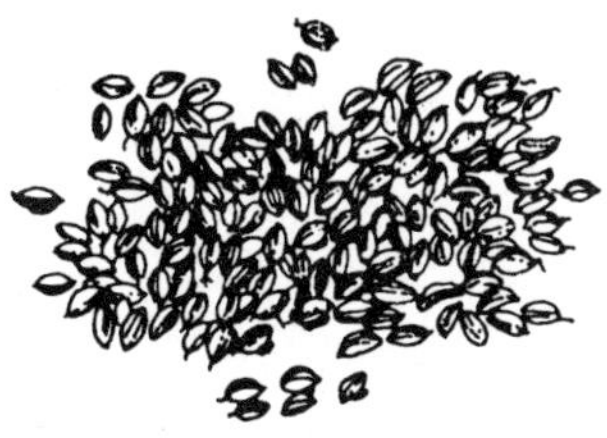

Ajwain was traditionally used for the treatment of a number of ailments: dyspepsia, diarrhoea, flatulence, indigestion, spasmodic disorders, microbial infections, etc. It has well known anti-parasitical properties.

As Medicine:

- Loss of appetite: Mix and powder equal quantities of ajwain, saunf, ginger and salt. Mix a teaspoon of this mixture in boiled rice along with ghee and eat thrice a day.
- Colic pains, indigestion, gas : Grind 2 tsp each ajwain and dried ginger into a fine powder. Add a little black salt. Take 1 tsp of this mixture with 1 teacup warm water frequently.
- Kidney- pain, renal colic: Mix and grind 1 tbsp black cumin, 2 tsp ajwain and 1 tsp black salt into a fine powder. Add 1 tsp brown vinegar. Take 1 tsp of this mixture every hour till symptoms subside.
- Nasal congestion in children: Crush a fistful of ajwain and tie up in a cotton napkin and place it near the pillow.
- Common cold, congestion in chest: Boil $^1/_2$ tsp ajwain along with 1 pinch of turmeric powder, in half a cup of water. Cool. Add 1 tsp honey and drink. Inhale vapours of ajwain boiling in a pan of water.
- Cough: Mix $^1/_2$ tsp ajwain seeds, 2 cloves and a pinch of salt. Powder and sip with a little warm water frequently.
- Respiratory problem due to blockage of dried phlegm: Crush 2 tsp ajwain seeds. Mix in a glass of buttermilk and drink.

CUMIN (*Jeera*)

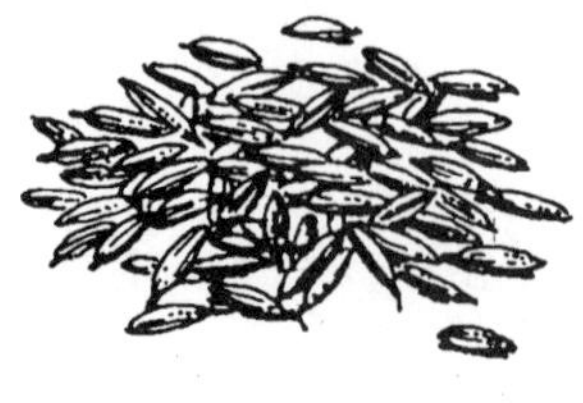

The seeds contains between 2.5 and 4.5 percent essential oils, the principal component of which is cumaldehyde. The oil is used in perfumery, for flavouring a variety of liquors, and used for medicinal purposes.

As Medicine:

- Diabetes: Take $^1/_2$ tsp of crushed jeera with water twice daily.
- Constipation, indigestion: Add equal quantities of jeera, black pepper dried ginger and dried curry leaves and powder them together. Add a little salt to taste. Add this mixture to hot ghee and eat with steamed rice.
- Gas, nausea: Mix equal quantities of jeera, black pepper and ginger. Make an infusion by boiling it in some water. Drink thrice a day for a few days.
- Heaviness in stomach, indigestion: Mix $^1/_4$ tsp each powdered jeera and black pepper in a glass of buttermilk. Drink two or three times a day for 2-3 days.
- Fatigue: Mix $^1/_2$ tsp each jeera, coriander seeds, black pepper and tuvar dal. Boil in water and drink with salt to taste.
- Insomnia: Mix 1 tsp powder of roasted jeera with a mashed ripe banana. Eat after dinner regularly.

CARDAMOM (*Ilaichi*)

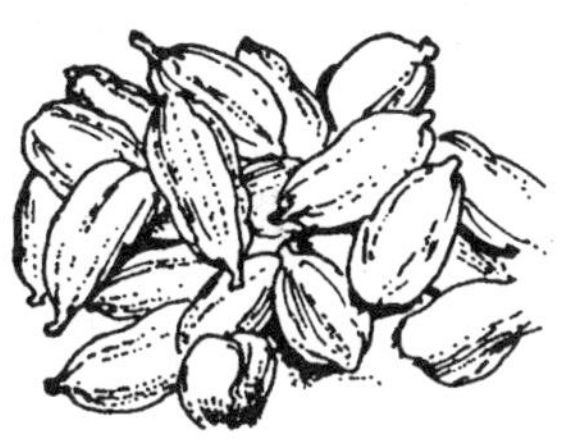

Cardamom (ılaichi) is used chiefly for relieving flatulence or feeling of dyspepsia, i.e. to promote digestion. It is administered with purgatives and as a flavouring agent. Powdered with cloves and ginger, it is good in indigestion. In ancient times, the dried seeds were used in asthma, bronchitis, piles, diseases of the bladder, headache, earache and toothache, as a breath freshener and energy booster.

As Medicine:

- Dyspepsia, nausea and loss of taste: Make a decoction of mint leaves and powdered cardamom seeds and drink.
- Indigestion: Make a fine powder of 1 tsp each cardamom seeds and saunf. Take $^{1}/_{4}$ tsp with water, twice daily, after meals.
- Bad breath of halitosis: Make an infusion of 1 tsp each cardamom, cinnamon and bay leaves in 1 teacup water. Drink it.
- Hoarseness, pharyngitis and sore throat: Boil 1 tsp each cinnamon and cardamom in a glass of water. Filter and use as a gargle when warm.
- Cough and cold: Mix seeds of cardamom along with 1 tbsp honey. Eat every day.
- Phlegmatic (with mucous) cough: Pour 1 teacup boiling water over $^{1}/_{2}$ tsp each ginger powder, clove powder and cinnamon powder. Filter. Sweeten with 1 tsp honey and drink.
- Diarrhoea, dysentery and exhaustion: Boil $^{1}/_{2}$ tsp powdered seeds as a weak tea and drink.

CLOVE (*Laung*)

Cloves (laung), which are the dried flower buds of the tree, are strongly aromatic, stimulant, and carminative. They are useful in flatulence and indigestion and stop nausea and vomiting. Clove oil is used as antiseptic and preservative. Taken internally, it is carminative and antispasmodic.

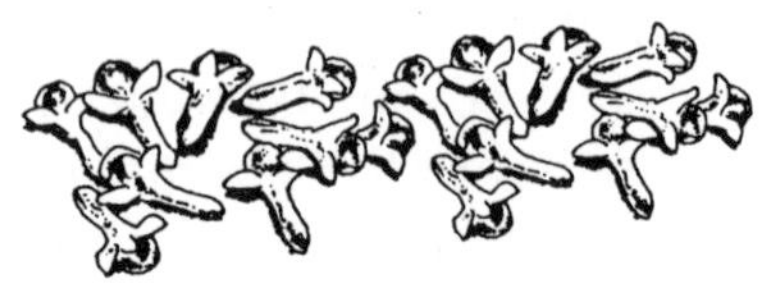

Cloves were used as a breath sweetener, a comforter for heart, liver, stomach and bowels; a remedy for nausea, colic, flatulence, toothache, and diarrhoea; a preventive for paralysis of the tongue; inflammation of the gums and loosening of the teeth. Rose water flavoured with cloves is a favourite eyewash.

It is a good anaesthetic for toothaches, a digestive aid and kills intestinal parasites.

As Medicine:

- Muscular cramps: Apply clove oil on the affected areas.
- Cholera: Drink a decoction of cloves regularly.
- Nausea: Chew a clove.
- Gum ailments, teeth ailments: Powder of roasted cloves is mixed in 1 teacup lukewarm water and used for gargling frequently.
- Headache: Make a smooth paste of cloves, water and salt. Apply on the temples (sides).
- Heaviness in head due to cough and cold: Grind 2 to 3 cloves into a fine paste along with $^1/_2$ tsp dried ginger and apply on nose and forehead.

- Toothache: Soak a piece of cotton wool in few drops of clove oil. Press on the affected tooth. Crush a clove and put it on the affected tooth.
- Throat irritation due to coughing: Chew 1 or 2 cloves.
- Bronchial afflictions: Boil 6 to 8 cloves in 1 cup water. A teaspoon of this decoction to be taken with honey frequently.

CINNAMON (*Dalchini*)

Cinnamon (dalchini) oil is used mostly as a flavouring agent in medicine. The bark of the stem and the oil obtained from it are useful as antiseptics, astringents and carminatives; the oil obtained from the leaves is used as a flavouring agent and for local application on certain rheumatic pains. It is commonly used as a condiment. It cures gastric debility and flatulence; and also has the property of destroying certain germs and fungi.

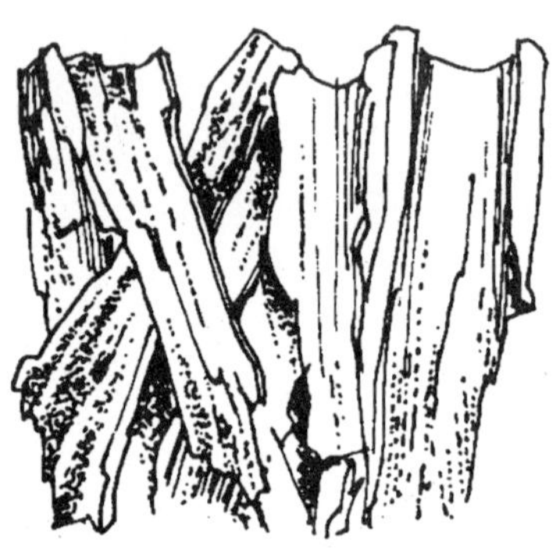

As Medicine:

- Diarrhoea: Combine 1 tsp each powdered ginger, cumin and cinnamon with honey and make into a thick paste. Take 1 tsp thrice daily.
- Bad breath: Boil 1 tsp cinnamon in 1 teacup water. Cool. Use frequently as a mouthwash.
- Loss of taste sensitivity in the tongue: Rub on the tongue a mixture of finely powdered cinnamon and honey and allow it to remain for sometime.
- Headache, caused by exposure to cold air: Mix 1 tsp finely ground cinnamon in 1 tsp water and apply on the affected parts.

- Cough: prepare a tea with $^1/_2$ tsp ginger, $^1/_4$ tsp cinnamon and 1 clove per cup of water. Sweeten with 1 tsp honey and drink.
- Acne, blackheads and pimples: Mix finely ground cinnamon powder in 1 tsp lime juice and apply on affected areas frequently.
- To improve the complexion: Add a pinch of cinnamon powder to $^1/_2$ tsp honey and apply on the face. Let it dry then wash it with water.
- To improve memory: Take a mixture of 1 tsp honey and a pinch of finely powdered cinnamon every night regularly.
- Sleeplessness: Boil $^1/_2$ tsp cinnamon in 1 teacup water for 5 minutes, strain and sweeten with honey. Take at bedtime.

NUTMEG (*Jaiphal*)

Jaiphal contains 7% to 14% essential oils. The oils are used as condiments and carminatives and to scent soaps and perfumes. It aids in relieving pain, abdominal swelling, indigestion and diarrhoea.

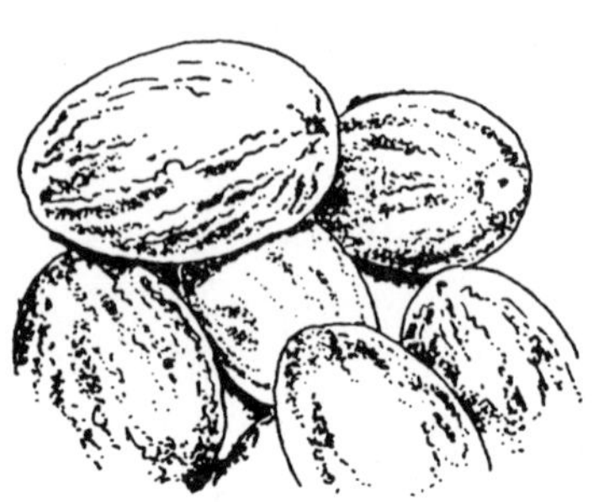

As Medicine:

- Colicky pain and diarrhoea: Take $^1/_8$ tsp finely ground nutmeg along with 1 tsp jaggery and 1 tsp ghee.
- Dehydration due to diarrhoea particularly in cholera: Soak half a nutmeg in 2-teacups water for over 2-3 hours. Mix equal quantities of this infusion and fresh coconut water. Drink twice or thrice daily.
- Diarrhoea: Add a pinch of nutmeg powder and $^1/_4$ tsp ginger paste to 1 glass buttermilk and drink.
- Dysentery: Take a pinch of powdered nutmeg with a cup of hot milk.
- Eczema, ringworm: Rub a nutmeg against a smooth stone slab with a little water and make a paste. Apply on the affected parts.
- Pimples: Grind equal quantities of nutmeg, black pepper and sandalwood and apply frequently.

TAMARIND (*Imli*)

Tamarind or imli contains vitamin C, iron and other minerals. It is a tonic and rejuvenative very useful in preventing and curing scurvy. The pulp of the ripe fruit is used in acute constipation and liver disorders like jaundice. Tamarind pulp has laxative properties; its infusion in water is a very refreshing, carminative drink; it is useful in fevers. Good for acute bronchitis, laryngitis, and whooping cough.

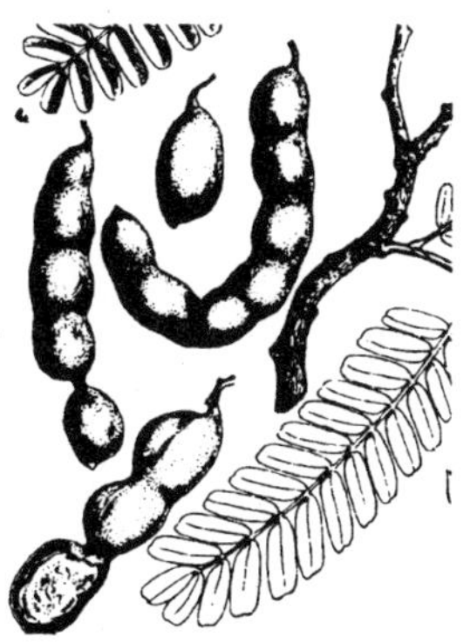

As Medicine:

- Blood clot/swelling due to injuries: After removing the seeds and fibre, mix the pulp (3tbsp) with 1 tsp salt and $^1/_2$ cup water. Mix thoroughly and heat the mixture in a container. When bearably hot, apply on the affected areas. Wash with water the next day and repeat for 3 days.
- Indigestion, loss of appetite, tastelessness: Rasam, a soup of tomato with tamarind pulp, cumin, coriander seeds, black pepper, curry leaves, ginger and garlic, either drunk straight or with plain, steamed rice.
- Fevers: Make an infusion of 1 tsp fruit pulp in 1 cup water and drink.
- Sore throat: Dilute the pulp with warm water and gargle.

HOLY BASIL (*Tulsi*)

The leaves and seeds of the plant are medicinal. They are used as a disinfectant, an immune stimulant, for intestinal parasites, for the stomach, lungs, spleen, and large intestines.

The juice or infusion of the leaves is useful in bronchitis, cataract and digestive complaints; is applied locally on ringworm and other skin diseases; is dropped in ears to relieve earache. A decoction of leaves is used to cure common colds. Seeds are useful in complaints of urinary system. Decoction of root is given in malarial fever to bring about sweating.

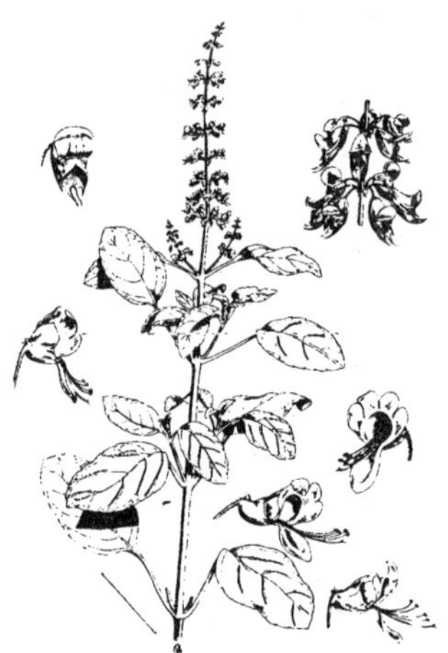

As Medicine:

- Liver Problems: Clean 10-15 leaves with hot water and eat every morning. Wash it down with a glass of hot water.
- Colic: Grind 1 tbsp tulsi leaves in water to make a fine paste and apply around the navel and on the abdomen.
- Digestion problems, dysentery, gastro-enteritis and gas: A decoction of 15-20 tulsi leaves to be taken along with a pinch of rock salt.

- Fevers of unknown origin: Boil 1 tbsp leaves with 1 tsp powdered cardamom in 2 teacups water. Take 1 cup of this decoction with milk and sugar to taste, 2 or 3 times a day.
- Cold and cough: Tulsi leaves (15-20) to be frequently chewed with jaggery.
- Prevention of cold: 10 leaves boiled in 1 teacup milk. This is a recommended nutritive supplement for children.
- Ringworm: Grind finely a bunch of leaves and apply on the cleaned affected area.
- Cardiac pain, cold, influenza, low blood pressure, pain in ribs, skin, diseases, worms, urinary diseases: Juice of leaves (10-15) mixed with 1 tsp honey to be taken daily in the morning.

TURMERIC (*Haldi*)

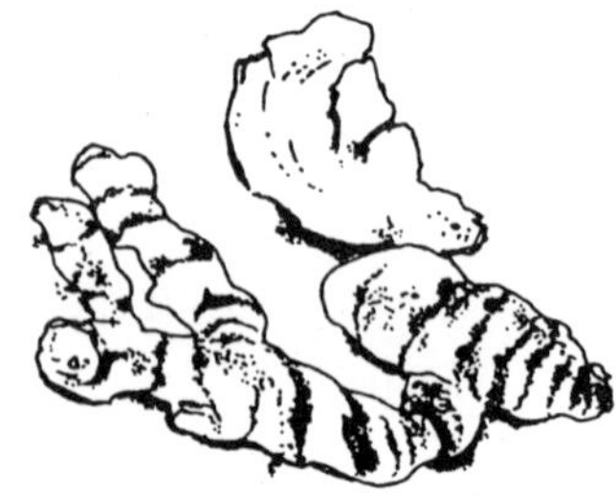

Turmeric or haldi is a root from the ginger family. It is an ideal disinfectant and an internal antiseptic. It arrests cholesterol problems, eliminates toxins and cools down the digestive and circulatory systems.

As Medicine:

- Muscle strain: Heat ginger paste with turmeric paste (1:1) and apply. Intestinal worms: Take $^{1}/_{4}$ tsp turmeric along with a glass of hot water 2 or 3 times daily.
- Common cold and blocked nose: Add 1 tbsp turmeric powder to boiling water. Inhale the vapours.
- Dry cough and sore throat: Drink a pinch of turmeric powder in a cup of hot milk at bedtime.
- Common cold: Mix 1 tsp turmeric powder along with $^{1}/_{4}$ tsp ajwain powder in 3 teacups hot water. Allow to cool. Take 1 tsp of this decoction along with 1 tsp honey twice daily for a few days.
- Acne, wounds, boils, tropical skin diseases: Make a paste of equal quantities of turmeric and sandalwood powder in water and apply. Cracks in the soles, itching, skin infection: Finely grind equal quantities of turmeric and neem leaves and apply on the affected areas.

FENNEL (*Saunf*)

Saunf is an excellent stomach and intestinal remedy and also a diuretic. Its decoction is given to the infants for colic and flatulence.

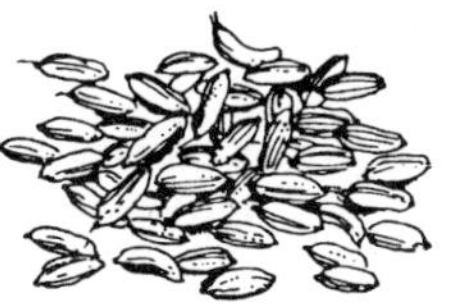

As Medicine:

- Anaemia: Boil 6 tsp each crushed saunf and red rose petals in 1½ teacup water and strain. Take twice daily.
- Indigestion and gas: Have roasted saunf daily after meals.
- Constipation: Make a very fine powder of 1 tsp each of the following: saunf, dried ginger and rock salt. Take 1 tsp with water at bedtime.
- Diarrhoea: Grind 3 tsp ginger along with 5 tsp saunf into a fine powder. Add enough honey to make a thick paste. Take 1 tsp in tea three times daily.
- Colic: Boil 1 tbsp saunf in a glass of milk for 10 minutes. Strain and drink. Drink 1 teacup decoction of rose water with honey and saunf.

CURRY LEAVES (*Meethi Neem*)

Curry leaves popularly known as meethi Neem are a must in the south-Indian cuisine. These leaves increase the appetite, eliminate body heat and generally strengthen the body.

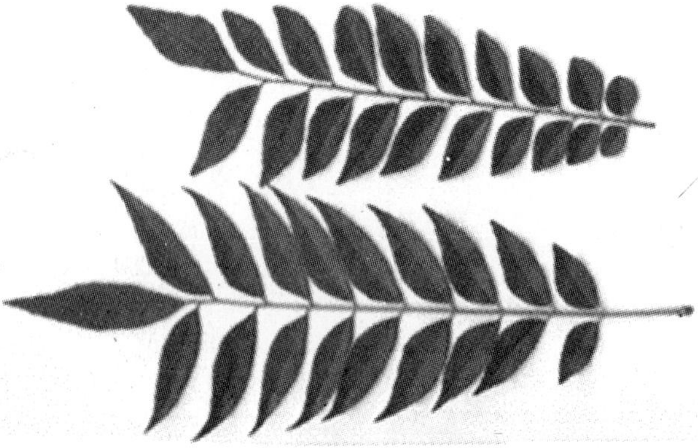

As Medicine:

- Diabetes due to hereditary factors, obesity: Eat 10 fresh curry leaves every morning for 3 to 4 months. (Avoid fatty foods, sweets and alcohol)
- Diarrhoea, dysentery and piles: Mix juice of 15-20 tender leaves with 1 tsp honey and drink.
- Nausea, indigestion and stomach upset: Make a chutney of a handful of fresh leaves by adding 1 tsp tamarind, one fried red chilli and salt to taste. Eat with food. Extract juice from 15 to 20 curry leaves and mix it with buttermilk. Take twice or thrice daily.
- Burns: Apply curry leaves as poultices over affected areas.

CORIANDER (*Dhania*)

Dhania or coriander kills bacteria, fungi and is good on cuts and wounds to kill micro-organisms. Coriander is useful for anyone who has a battle with gastric ulcers and other symptoms of acidity.

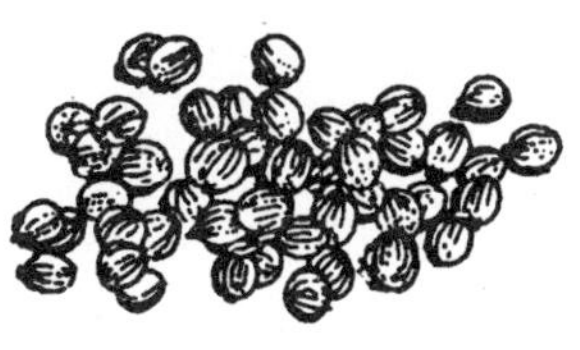

As Medicine:

- Swellings: Drink coriander tea (1 tsp coriander seeds steeped in a cup of warm water).
- High cholesterol: Regular intake of coriander decoction made by boiling 2 tsp dry seed powder in 1 teacup water.
- Diarrhoea: 2 to 3 tsp coriander seeds soaked overnight in water and taken next morning with 1 cup buttermilk.
- Mouth ulcers: Boil 1 tsp coriander seeds in 2 teacups water till it is reduced to 1 teacup. Add sugar to taste and drink when lukewarm. Repeat twice or thrice a day.
- Anaemia and kidney problems: Frequent intake of coriander tea: boil or steep 2 tsp coriander powder in a glass of water. Add sugar to taste.

FENUGREEK (*Methi*)

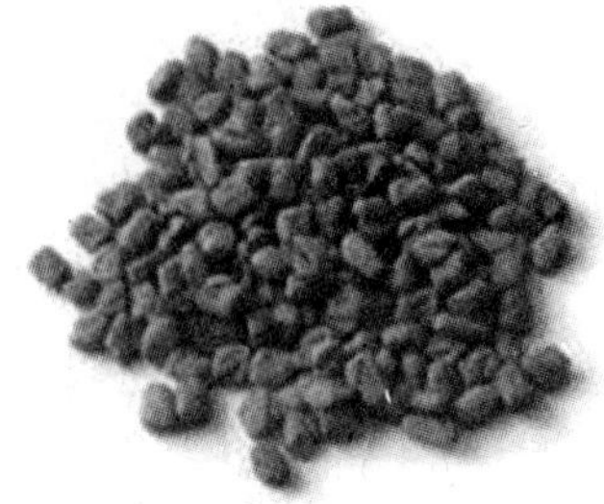

Reduces mucous in sinus and asthmatic conditions. It lowers cholesterol. These seeds make excellent tea for intestinal irritation or as a gargle tea for sore throats. It can also be ground as a poultice for wounds or inflamed areas.

As Medicine:

- Cardiac problems: Boil 1 tsp methi seeds in 1¼ cups water. Strain and add 2 tsp honey. Take twice daily.
- Diabetes: 2 tsp powdered seeds taken daily with milk. The treatment should continue for at least a month.
- Hypo-function of liver, indigestion: Allow the seeds to sprout and eat with breakfast.
- Dysentery: Soak 2 tsp methi seeds in coconut water or in buttermilk for a few hours. Strain and drink.
- Pain during urination, stomachache: Mix ¼ tsp powdered seeds in buttermilk and drink.
- Fever, body odour and mouth odour: Tea made by boiling 1 tsp methi seeds, to be taken twice or thrice a day.
- Baldness, falling hair: Grind methi seeds in water and apply on the head. Allow to soak for at least 40 minutes before washing. Repeat every morning for a month.
- Boils, ulcers and sores: Grind seeds into a paste and apply on the affected parts.

TO EAT SALT OR NOT

Since ancient times human beings have highly valued salt. But now medical opinion says we could be better off to give it up completely.

The chemical name of common salt is sodium chloride. It is an important constituent of our blood (0.9gm%). Sodium helps in the conduction of nerve impulses, contraction of muscles and maintaining the water balance in the body. It also plays an important role in the regulation of acid-base balance in the body fluids including blood, lymph, tears and gastrointestinal secretions. Chloride is an important component of blood plasma and also helps in the formation of hydrochloric acid in the stomach for digestion. But all this requires only a total intake of 5gm salt in a day!

Under normal circumstances, there is some salt present in every natural food we eat, which is enough to meet our body's daily requirement. However during summer or while exerting, the requirement of salt increases, which if not fulfilled, might result in muscle cramps, irritability and general apathy. We must also remember here that in addition to natural foods we are consuming salt (especially sodium as preservative) in various processed foods such as soft drinks, sauces, confectionary, pasta, tinned/canned foods, butter, cheese, pickles, cornflakes etc.

Soviet specialists prescribe 'no salt' diets for people who have diseases of heart and kidney. They have found that even some common ailments like bronchitis and skin eruptions are helped, by giving up salt. The theory seems that, giving up salt relieves the kidneys, heart and even certain glands, from the chemical work of forever removing excess salts out of the body via urine.

Excess of salt is also found to interfere with the elimination of certain wastes from the body like uric acid and therefore contributing indirectly to diseases like gout.

Japanese use salt very heavily and their death rate from strokes (due to high blood pressure) is extremely high. Natives of South Pacific, who eat no salt ever, almost never have high blood pressure or strokes. Negroes in the USA, are heavy salt takers, and have three times more blood pressure problems than Whites in the same areas.

So the doctors have concluded that if every one went on a low salt diet, blood pressure diseases would fall by 50%. This is very important since these diseases kill far more people even today than does cancer.

Are some people free from blood pressure problems because they do not eat salt, or because they lead quiet, stress-free lives? Though it is true that if you have certain heart or kidney diseases, salt can be harmful, but does salt cause high blood pressure? Or, is the main cause stress?

Doctors claim that only a small section of the population is harmed by surplus salt. In their view, individual human beings differ greatly in their 'response' to salt. Physical exercise (labour, sports) profoundly affects the average person's response to salt. Perhaps inactive people do not 'handle' it well.

There is a theory that says that the overweight people can bring down their blood pressure by only reducing weight. Now there is yet another theory, which says, that reducing salt intake helps in weight reduction.

Now in this confusion of whether salt is good or bad, the best would be to go off salt for two weeks. If you feel better, keep it up. The minute you feel week, go back to your salt cellar, but don't over do it. It might be a good idea to use rock salt (saindha namak) and black salt (kala namak) instead of table salt. For people with a history of high blood pressure, it is strongly advised to use potassium salt instead of the normal salt (sodium chloride).

CEREALS

Cereal grains are the seeds of domesticated grasses. They have been modified and improved by centuries of cultivation and selective breeding. In the rural areas of many countries cereals provide more than 70% of the energy in the diet. As one becomes more prosperous, this proportion falls, but cereals remain the staple item of the diet. Only isolated people, such as the Eskimos, are almost entirely carnivorous and do not cultivate cereals. The principal cereals are wheat, rice, maize, millets, barley, oats and rye.

The whole grains of all cereals have a similar chemical composition and nutritive value. They provide energy and also some protein, which is usually of good quality. They contain appreciable amounts of minerals like calcium, iron and phosphorus. Whole cereals are totally devoid of vitamin C and practically devoid of vitamin A activity. Yellow maize is the only cereal containing significant amounts of carotene (gets converted to vitamin A in our body). Whole cereal grains also contain useful amounts of the B group vitamins. Germination enhances the vitamin B complex levels and produces vitamin C in the cereal grains.

If your meal is rich in whole grain cereals, you may be rest assured about the carbohydrate, protein, vitamin B complex and fibre levels of your diet.

WHEAT (*Gehun*)

Wheat is the most widely used cereal in the world. In order to make wheat flour the coarser part of the grain (bran) is removed and the white flour remains. The whiter the flour, the lower is its nutritive value. Wheat bran or 'chokar' contains a large proportion of proteins, vitamins and of course fibre. Wheat also has a high gluten content, which is what makes the bread rise. Gluten is a tough, sticky, nitrogenous substance that forms mucous and coats the villi of the intestines. If the villi get too heavily coated, nutrients cannot be absorbed, resulting in malabsorption. This also affects the myelin sheath of nerves. Wheat products should be consumed in moderation or not at all if you suffer from intestinal disorders.

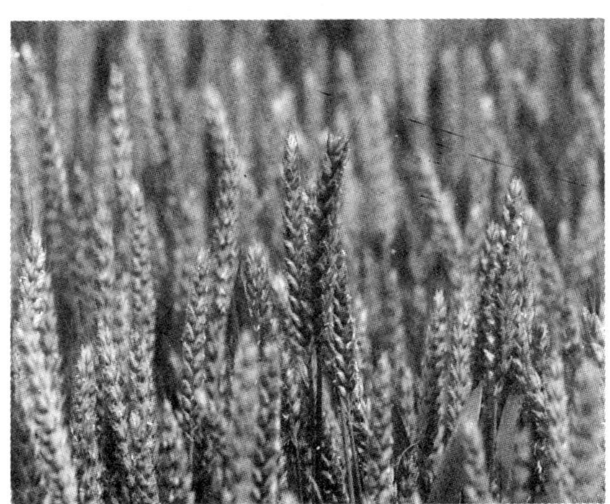

As Medicine:

- Poultice of warm wheat dough is used to treat boils and swellings on the body.
- Wheat sprouts are known to control blood sugar levels.
- Wheat bran contains a tumour inhibiting substance, which taken regularly, prevents the chances of cancer.

RICE (*Chawal*)

Rice is rich in starch, moderate in proteins, and poor in fat, iron and calcium. There are four forms of rice: brown rice, parboiled, regular milled and pre-cooked. It comes in short, medium, and long grained varieties. Brown rice is high in all the B vitamins, calcium, phosphorus, iron and protein. It keeps the blood sugar stabilized so you do not feel hungry for longer periods and, therefore, you eat less often. Brown rice is the easiest grain to digest, making it good for those with food allergies. Milled rice loses some of its nutrients, though parboiled rice has its nutrients better preserved. Parboiling involves boiling the paddy in water. After draining off the water, this paddy is dried and milled. Researches have indicated that a low-fat diet including fibre from rice bran can reduce cholesterol levels by 15%.

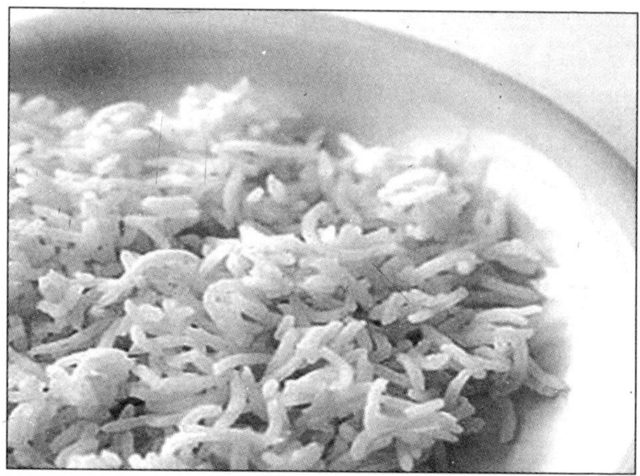

As Medicine:

- Water of boiled rice is effective in curing diarrhoea, dysentery and nausea.
- Boiled rice taken as a daily staple helps in reducing obesity.

BARLEY (*Jau*)

Barley was once much used as a human food (now used only in the form of barley water for the sick!). It is widely grown in almost all parts of the world. It produces the most satisfactory malt for brewers and is the basis of the best beers and whisky. This grain is rich in potassium, sulphur and phosphorus. Barley stimulates the liver and lymphatic system, enhancing the discharge of toxic waste from the body.

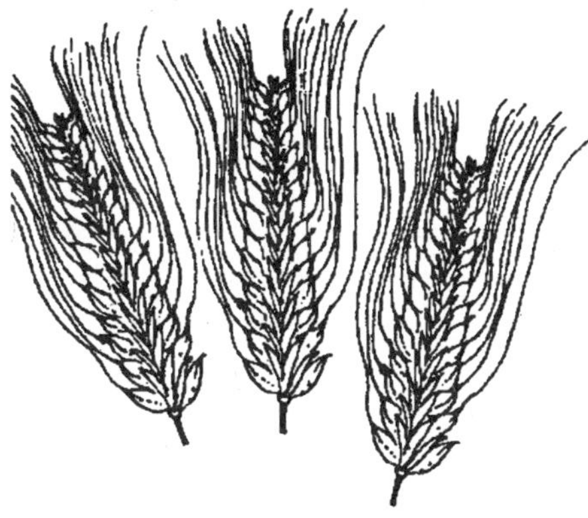

Barley aids the suppression of cholesterol production in the liver and also prevents dietary fats and cholesterol from being absorbed in the intestines.

As Medicine:

- Barley sprouts are full of energy and should be taken regularly by people indulging in strenuous work or bodybuilding exercises.
- Juice of barley sprouts helps to cure arthritis.
- Barley flour mixed with wheat flour in the chapatis is seen to reduce the blood cholesterol levels.

MILLET (*Bajara*)

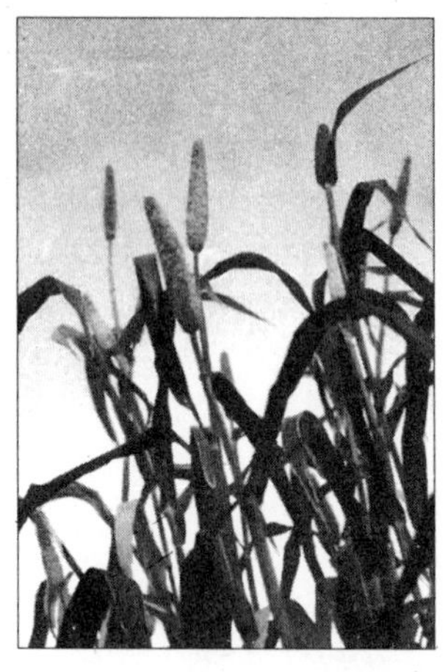

Millet, the cheapest of all cereals, has always been regarded as a poor man's food. Although this is understandable, for it has a good nutritive value. There are a number of varieties of millets, having an even greater variety of names–jowar, cholam, ragi, bajra, cambu, madua, to name a few. Millets are high in carbohydrates, with protein content varying from 6 to 11 per cent and fat varying from 1. 5 to 5 per cent. They are somewhat strong in taste and cannot be made into leavened bread but are mainly consumed in flatbreads and porridges or prepared and eaten much like rice. The grains are also used in making edible oil, starch, dextrose (a sugar), and alcoholic beverages.

It is the only grain that because of its alkaline nature is good for the spleen, pancreas, and stomach and benefits those who suffer from acidosis, colitis, ulcers and urinary disorders.

As Medicine:

- A regular intake of millets in any form keeps a check on the deposits of any kind of fats in the body.
- Millets have significant amounts of iron, lecithin, and choline, which help keep cholesterol in check and stop the formation of certain types of gallstones.

CORN (*Makai*)

Maize or 'Makai' is also known as 'corn' in India and 'Indian corn' in the United States. Unlike other cereals, maize is mostly consumed without milling, which helps it to retain all the nutrients. Corn is one of the easiest foods to digest. It is very high in roughage. For those who want to avoid weight gain, corn should be used sparingly because it is rich in carbohydrates. Yellow corn is very high in magnesium, which is a wonderful bowel regulator. It is a great bone and muscle builder. Yellow corn is also rich in phosphorus, which makes it an excellent food for the brain and nervous system.

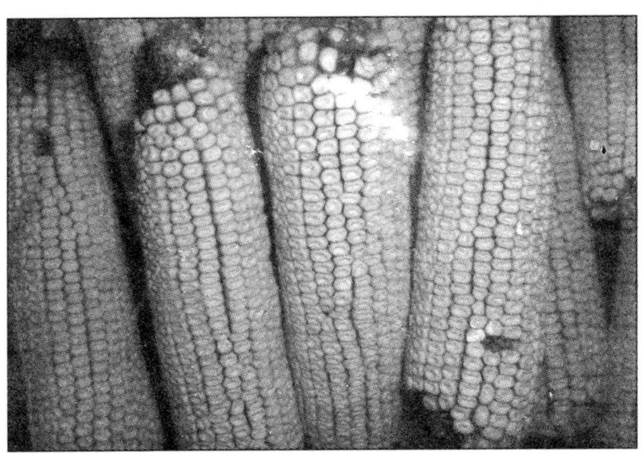

As Medicine:

- Paste of coarse cornflour in water acts as an effective face pack to remove acne and other skin blemishes.
- Corn grains consumed daily help to keep a check on the blood cholesterol levels.

OATS (*Jai*)

Oats and oat flour have the ability to normalize blood glucose in diabetes. They are good for a slow working thyroid. Oats contain the highest amount of fat of all grains creating warmth and stamina in the body. Oats retain more food value than wheat processing. The protein content in oats is easily assimilated and helps neutralize excess cholesterol. It contains high amounts of calcium, iodine, phosphorus, iron, vitamin E and the whole B complex. Oats are the most acidic of cereals and have a high gluten content.

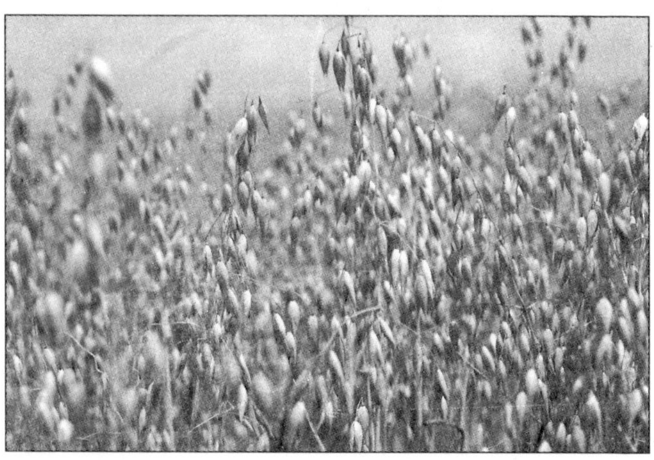

As Medicine:

- Oats taken regularly in breakfast help to control the levels of sugar and triglycerides in the blood, and hence prevent the risk of heart attacks.
- Oat-flour paste in honey, applied on the skin is effective in removing acne, blackheads or any other skin blemishes.

PULSES

Pulses or dals are capable of surviving all sorts of climates and soils, and so are cultivated in almost all civilized parts of the world. Thus, there are very few people to whose diet pulses do not make some regular contribution.

The most common or popular pulses in our country are Black gram (Urad), Green gram (Moong), Red gram (Arhar), Bengal gram (Chana), Red kidney bean (Rajmah), Soya bean, Lentil (Masoor), etc. A pulse known as Khesri dal was once sown widely in Central India. Its special value was that it was very resistant to drought. Even if the main cereal crop failed in a dry season, some Khesri dal could always be harvested. However, it is found that if a large amount of Khesri dal is eaten, paralysis of lower limbs, known as Lathyrism is commonly followed.

In Western countries, amongst pulses, beans and peas are more popular than our usual dals. Baked beans are very popular in Western countries, and have now come to India as well. Like Soya bean, the other beans can also be used to enhance the nutritive value of the diet.

All pulses (including beans) supply the same amount of calories as cereals, i.e., 100 calories per ounce (30g). The protein content is 20-25g%, about twice as much as cereals. Pulses are deficient in methionine (an amino acid), but are rich in lysine, an amino acid in which many cereals are deficient. Thus a cereal-pulse-protein combination has a nutritive value as good as animal protein. That is why pulses have been described as 'the poor man's meat'! Dal-roti, khichdi, idli, dosa, etc. are excellent examples of complete protein. The fat content of pulses is negligible, about 1-2g%.

Pulses are a good source of B complex vitamins. Also, there are no milling losses as there are in cereals. Although pulses like cereals are deficient in vitamin C, yet this can be taken care of by germinating them. Sprouted pulses become an excellent source of vitamin C. On germination, the vitamin A content of the pulses can also be increased–third day after germination, when the shoots change from yellow to green.

The iron content of most pulses is high, being 8-10mg%—making them an ideal food for the anaemics (not the only food though).

Groundnuts/peanuts, in fact, are also in the family of pulses, and not of nuts! They resemble the other pulses in general nutritive value, except that they are rich in fat. The whole seed contains about 40% fat, twice the amount in Soya bean.

It is believed, that Black gram and Lentil, when germinated contain a growth promoting factor–nature not yet known. Apart from these features, pulses, in any case, enhance the nutritive value of any diet, and therefore its intake in our daily diet should be encouraged. A katori of dal should not be looked down upon!

RED KIDNEY (*Rajmah*)

Rajmah or Red kidney beans are very popular the world over as a main dish or even in salads and soups. They are rich in all nutrients, protein and fibre. They are the richest in fibre of all the pulses.

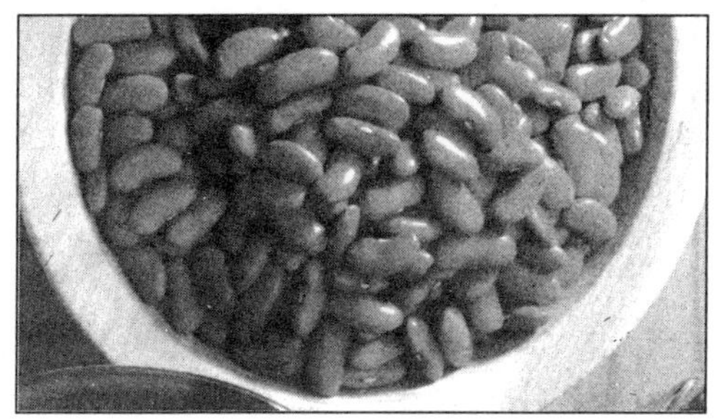

SOYA BEANS

The soya bean is valued for its high protein content, but it also has an exceptionally high amount of other vitamins and minerals. Soya bean oil is excellent for frying, is easily digestible, and contains no cholesterol. It also rejuvenates the endocrine glands.

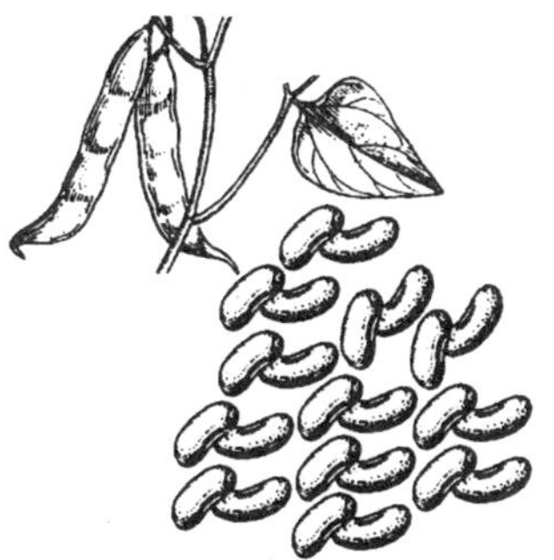

BENGAL GRAM (*Choley*)

Bengal gram contains Niacin, a vitamin mainly known and acclaimed for its ability to prevent Pellagra, a disease that is characterized by gastrointestinal distur-bances and skin lesions. Interestingly, it has been seen that a regular consumption of Bengal gram over a period of several weeks reduces cholesterol!

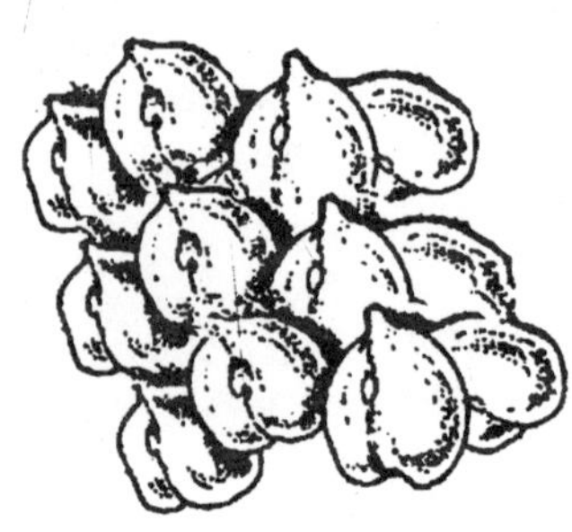

Pulses as Medicine:

- Germinated whole pulses are an age-old remedy in weakness, fatigue, and general debility.
- The water in which any dal is boiled gives relief in fevers, respiratory and urinary disorders.
- Whole pulses ground and added to the wheat flour help to improve the protein and fibre content of the chapatis, which helps in keeping a check on the blood sugar and cholesterol levels.
- Face packs of ground pulses in curd are effective skin toners.
- Poultices of coarsely ground soaked pulses are used to treat skin abscesses.

NUTS

A nut is an edible seed or kernel enclosed in a hard shell. The nuts are rich in proteins, fats, carbohydrates, minerals and vitamin B complex. Their food value may be high but, as medicine only almonds and coconut are popular.

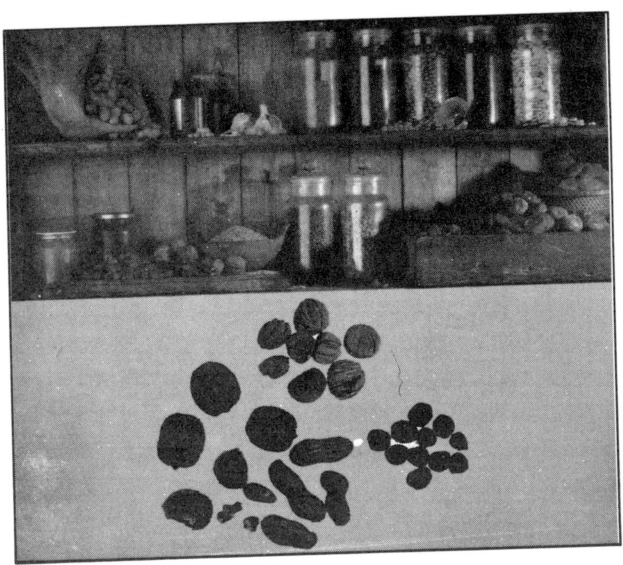

ALMOND (*Badam*)

Almonds provide small amounts of protein, iron, calcium, phosphorus, and B vitamins and are high in fat. They may be eaten raw, blanched, or roasted.

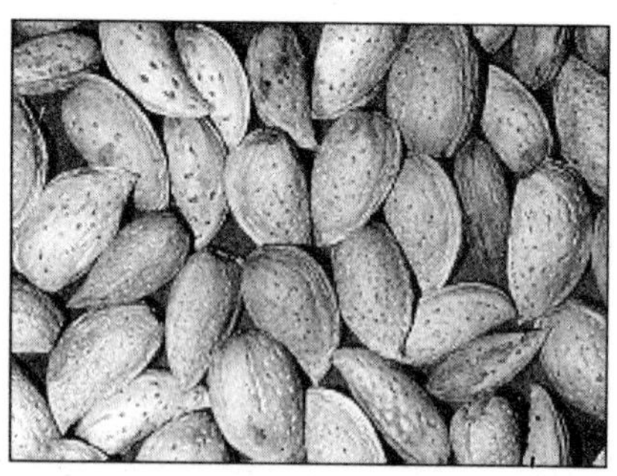

As Medicine:

- Constipation: Grind separately 5 almonds and 5 dried dates. Combine them and add 10 tsp honey. Take 3 tsp of this mixture twice daily.
- Sore throat and cough: Soak 2-3 almonds and 1 dried fig for a few hours in 1 cup water. Remove the outer skins and grind everything together into a paste. Add 1 tbsp honey and eat at bedtime.
- Yellowing of teeth, toothache: Burn the shells of almonds and powder. Use as toothpowder.
- Psoriasis, skin problems: Powder a few almonds and boil thoroughly in water. Apply this paste on affected areas and let it remain overnight. Next morning wash it off with water.
- Help in maintaining a good complexion: Soak 10 almonds overnight in water. After discarding the outer skin, grind the kernels along with a little milk (or malai) into a very fine paste. Apply daily (before taking a bath) on the exposed parts of body, i.e. face, neck, forearms legs, etc every day.

COCONUT (*Nariyal*)

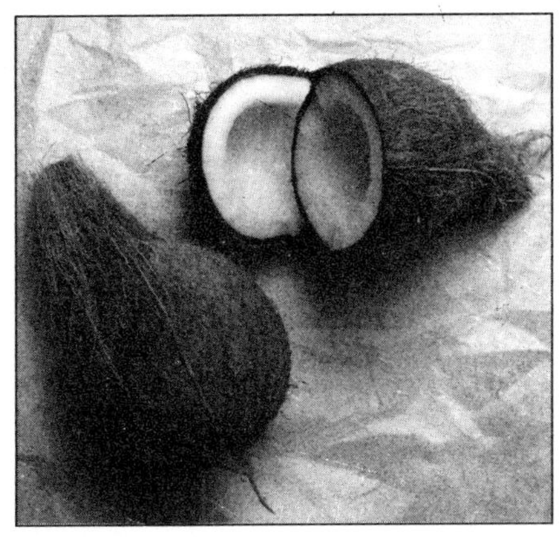

The liquid inside green nuts offers a refreshing drink during hot summer months, which keeps the body cool. It prevents sunstroke, heat stroke and vomiting. It is given in thirst, fever and urinary disorders; is a blood purifier and checks motion sickness and nausea.

Coconut milk compares to mother's milk in its chemical balance. It is complete protein food when taken in its natural form.

As Medicine:

- Stomach ulcer: Frequently drink tender coconut water and milk extracted from the kernel.
- Mouth ulcers: Mix some coconut milk with honey and massage the gums 3 to 4 times a day. Gargle with freshly extracted coconut milk frequently.
- Thinning of hair: Bathe the hair with 1 teacup coconut milk twice or thrice a week for a few months.
- Prickly heat: Grind well 1 tbsp grated coconut along with 1 tsp cumin and apply the paste on the affected areas.
- Intestinal parasites: To prevent such infections, add coconut to the daily diet.

MILK

From the earliest dawn of the human history to the present day, the great value of milk as human food has always been recognized and there is evidence to show that the first occupation of mankind was cow keeping. There is no adequate substitute for milk. Milk, in fact is the only single article of food that represents a complete diet; it is excellent for the growing children and has no equal for the promotion of growth and nutrition. No food has a wider acceptability or offers a greater variety of uses. Think of all the lovely sweets and paneer products and ice creams.

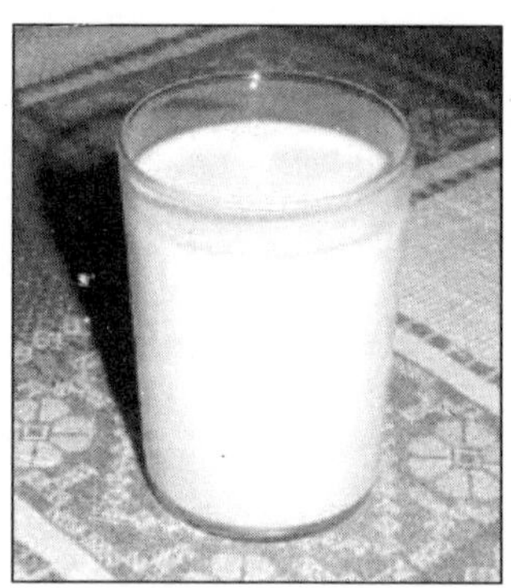

Milk is a complete substance containing almost all the nutrients. The exact composition of milk varies with the breed of the cattle and the food used. Also there are many types of milk, like the ass's, reindeer's, sheep's, goat's, camel's, mare's, yak's and even elephant's milk, apart from the mother's milk and the routine cow's milk and buffalo's milk. Here we will discuss the usual milk available in the market, be it cow's or buffalo's or any recognized dairy's.

Too many people become concerned about the energy or calorie value of milk and sometimes eliminate milk from their diets due to this reason. Actually the fat content of the milk determines the calorie provided by it. For example, the cow's milk contains half as much fat as contained by buffalo's milk, so the calories provided by the cow's milk are quite less, as compared to those provided by buffalo's milk. In case you are calorie-conscious, and want to drink milk yet avoid putting on weight, just remove the fat from the milk, simply skim off the 'malai' and there you are with a low calorie nutritious drink! The average protein content of milk is about 4%. Milk contains all the vitamins in appreciable amounts, except vitamin C, which is present in very little quantity. As far as minerals are concerned, it is well known that milk is a very good source of calcium and phosphorus, required for the growth and development of the bones. Apart from these, milk also contains other minerals like sodium, potassium and magnesium too, but very little iron. As a complete food, easily given, readily digested and absorbed, milk is an ideal food for invalids, especially for patients with acute illnesses and during convalescence. And in case you want to gain weight, the fatty preparations of the milk like butter and cream are very good for it.

But, with all this goodness, some people actually cannot tolerate milk! They may even have an allergy for it. Things like abdominal pain and discomfort, diarrhoea or even constipation may be caused by milk in some people. But there is nothing to worry about, as milk is not indispensable. It may be the sole food of the human infant for the first few months of life, but, after that, once the infant can eat other food items as well, milk ceases to be in the top position in the list of priorities. It has been shown that the children can grow well on a mixed diet composed of cereals, dals and vegetables with no milk. The individual nutrients provided by milk can be obtained from other dietary sources as well. The proteins are available in dals, the vitamins and minerals in fruits and vegetables. The calories are abundant in fats, oils and sugars.

Milk being a complete food and the rest of it, applies to the bacteria as well. They thrive beautifully in it and so we have the milk borne diseases, the commonest being typhoid, tuberculosis, cholera and dysentery.

CHEESE (*Paneer*)

The basic process in cheese making is the clotting of the milk.

Most processed cheeses contain 25 to 35 percent of protein and this protein is of high biological value. The fat content usually varies from 16 to 40 per cent. Cheese is also rich in calcium, vitamins A and B. Cottage cheese (paneer) contains 4 per cent fat.

CURD (*Dahi*)

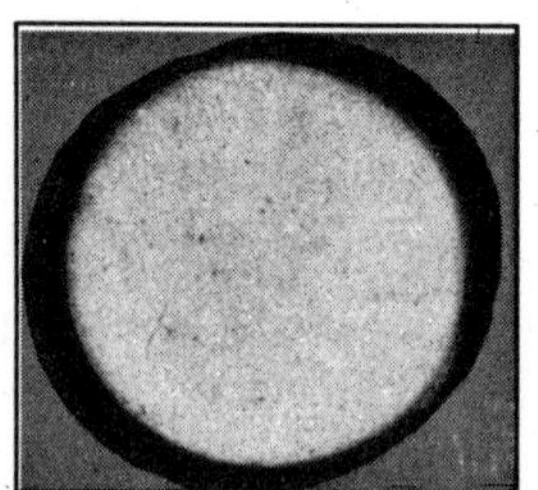

Made from milk, it has a custard-like consistency and a slight sour taste. It has a list of health benefits too long to mention and is important in the daily diet helping digestion and reducing bloating and gas. Curd is very high in the B-vitamins. It replenishes friendly bacteria in the intestinal tract that are vital to good health.

SUGARS

Sugars are of many types including cane sugar, beet sugar, maple sugar, corn sugar and palm sugar. The sugar commonly used is the cane sugar, sugarcane being the largest source of the sugar worldwide. Sugar is a relatively late arrival in the food scene. Initially the sweetening agent used to be honey. Sweet taste is highly relished by most of us, and sweets and desserts form an important part of any feast. The sweetening agent sugar is chemically known as sucrose.

"Sugar and spice, and everything nice..." goes the nursery rhyme. Questions are now being raised as to whether sugar is really all that nice. It is believed that the high consumption of sugar in western countries may be partly responsible for the high incidence of heart disease in those countries.

Apart from being popular amongst people, especially children, sugar also enjoys immense popularity in the bacterial community. Bacteria just love sugar and thrive beautifully in it. (If you also provide some air and water along with.) That is why high consumption of sugar and sweets is associated with a high incidence of dental caries or decay of teeth. The habit of eating sticky sweets like toffees and caramels very often leads to tooth decay, because particles of such sweets stick to the teeth enabling the bacteria to grow, flourish and destroy the teeth.

Due to economic considerations, administrators have classified sugar as an essential food commodity. On the other hand, a nutritionist would call sugar to be a non –

essential food, as its exclusion from the diet is harmless to man. Nutritionally speaking, the special function of sugar in the diet is providing energy, apart from imparting sweetness to the food. As far as the energy is concerned, it is also provided by rice, bread, that is the cereals, and pulses too. These food items also provide protein and vitamins along with energy. Even tubers like potatoes have a great deal of energy in them. In contrast, sugar supplies only energy and nothing else.

There are two commonly available varieties of sugar, namely white and brown sugar. The difference between the two of them is very simple. White sugar is the refined form of brown sugar.

As far as the food value is concerned, brown sugar is definitely better than the white one. White sugar certainly looks more attractive, especially in the form of cubes. But as they say, "beauty is skin deep", so is the case with white sugar. On the other hand, brown sugar, though has dull, deceptive appearance, and imparts a soiled look to the puddings, has certain good points hidden in it. Together with energy, brown sugar also gives us some iron and vitamin B complex. Iron is needed for the formation of blood, and the B vitamins help in digesting food. Jaggery, commonly known as "gur", is also a form of brown sugar and therefore, is better than white sugar.

So we see that sugar is not a very useful food, as it caters more to the palate than to health.

HONEY

Honey is a sweet thick fluid prepared by the honeybees from the nectar of flowers. Nutritionally speaking, honey contains about 75-80% sugar and the rest is a mixture of water and minerals like phosphorus, calcium, magnesium, some acids and enzymes. So we see that together with minerals, honey also gives us energy, about 300 to 320 calories per 100ml of honey. To put it simply, one teaspoonful of honey would give us about 15 to 16 calories.

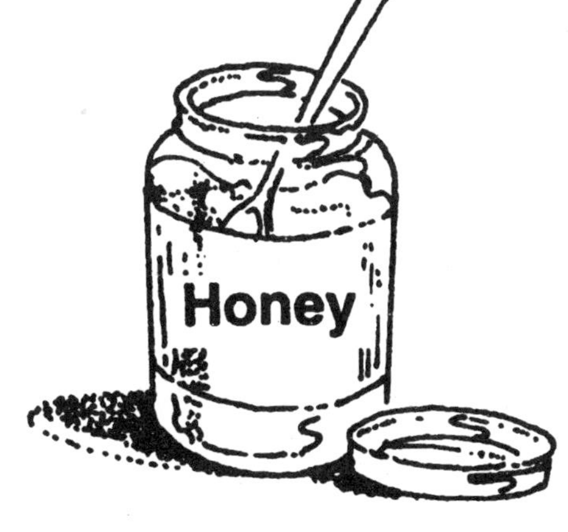

The enzymes present in honey aid in digestion of food especially raw sugars and starch. The difference between the commonly used sugar and honey is that, the sugars contained in honey are in very simple predigested forms and thus are directly absorbed by our body. Whereas the normal sugar has to be broken down in our body into simpler forms to be digested and absorbed. Apart from giving nutrition, honey can be used as a sweetening agent in sweets and desserts.

In addition to the excellent medicinal properties, honey is supposed to be a good thirst quencher. Arabs take honey and water across desserts. Another aspect of honey is its use in the beauty treatment. One of the most commonly used face packs for aging skin, is a mixture of honey and cornflour and limejuice.

So we see that honey is a pleasant, attractive, sweet item of food with plenty of other uses too. This does not mean that you can eat as much honey, as you like. We all know that excess of calories over and above what we require would make us fat and honey does have calories. Honey may improve your digestion but it should not be done at the cost of giving you a sweet tooth!

As Medicine:

- One to two teaspoonfuls of honey in a glass of hot milk is said to be a good sedative.
- For children the use of honey as a general tonic has been known from time immemorial. The reason being that honey acts as a disinfectant and an antiseptic. So a judicious internal administration of honey would render the digestive system aseptic and disease-causing germs would fail to thrive.
- Honey is good for sore throats, coughs and colds. An age-old cough mixture still used in many homes consists of honey and limejuice in equal parts.
- Honey is also reputed to be a good stimulant for a weak heart.
- As far as constipation is concerned, honey is a very popular laxative.

FATS AND OILS

Fats and oils are a valuable part of the diet, as they provide a concentrated source of energy and are also essential in cooking. They consist of mainly triglycerides. Vegetable oils and ghee have 9 calories per gram, but butter has less (about 7.3 calories per gram), as it contains some water.

Fats and oils provide not only energy but also essential fatty acids. However, they are not essential articles of diet. Oils and fats may be a source or potential source of fat-soluble vitamins. Most vegetable oils contain vitamin E. Corn oil contains small amounts of carotene (precursor of vitamin A). Animal fats contain vitamin D.

The minimal requirement of fats by the body is very low. But, for middle-aged people and sedentary workers, it should certainly not be more than 35% of their total energy intake.

High fat diets lead to obesity and contribute to a variety of diseases.

As Medicine:

Castor Oil

- Constipation: Take one teaspoonful of castor oil in warm milk at bedtime.
- Difficulty in urination: Take one teaspoonful of castor oil in warm water.

- Stomach colic: Mix castor oil and curd in equal quantities and drink the mixture. Repeat it after half an hour.
- Worms: Mix the castor oil and honey in equal amounts. Take one tablespoonful two times a day for three days.

Note: Only medicated castor oil is recommended for internal uses.

Coconut Oil

- Worms: Take two teaspoonfuls of the oil twice a day for five days.
- Whooping cough: Take two teaspoonfuls of oil three times a day. It gives relief immediately.
- Dandruff: Mix camphor powder in coconut oil. Apply it on the head rubbing with fingers at the roots of hair for 10 minutes. It will destroy dandruff and will also protect against baldness.

Warning: People suffering from asthma, bronchitis and influenza should totally avoid the internal use of coconut oil.

Mustard Oil

- Cough: Mix mustard oil and gur (jaggery) in equal amounts. Eat a teaspoonful of this mixture two times a day for three weeks.
- Toothache: Mix common salt and mustard oil. Apply it over the teeth and rub gently. It heals the pain of swollen gums and regular use gets rid of the bad breath.

TEA

Nobody knows exactly, where or when, the first cup of tea was brewed. According to folklore, Emperor ' Shen Nung' who reigned over China in 273 BC discovered the stimulating effect of tea accidentally when wild tea leaves fell into his pot of boiling drinking water. Chinese have probably been drinking tea in some form or the other since the fourth century AD and considering that wild tea grew in many parts of Assam, it is not unlikely that tea drinking in India too is as old as in China.

The raw material for tea manufacture normally consists of two young leaves and an unopened leaf bud - the famous 'two leaves and a bud' formula, but, plucking of longer shoots containing 3 or even 4 leaves is not uncommon. The freshly harvested tea shoots can be processed into the various kinds of tea, namely, black tea, green tea, oolong tea and instant tea. In the manufacture of black tea (the usual tea that we all drink), the material undergoes 'fermentation' while in the production of green tea, delicate and subtle in flavour, fermentation is purposely omitted. Oolong tea leaves get an intermediate treatment, considered to be 'semi-fermented'. Instant tea, like instant coffee, is a dehydrated product containing only the soluble constituents of tea.

There is hardly any drink that is not a food too, in terms of the calories it provides tea is no exception. A cup of tea, containing 2 tablespoonfuls of milk and a teaspoonful of sugar, yields about 40 calories. Milk contains casein, which makes the tannin in the tea insoluble, thus removing some of its astringency (acidic effect). Apart from the milk and sugar generally added, the tea infusion contains marginal quantities of vitamins and minerals, but no significant quantities of extractable proteins, carbohydrates or fats.

Tea is fairly rich in most of the B group vitamins. Apart from these, it is also a good source of vitamin E and K and Beta-carotene (changes into vitamin A in our body). Tea contains traces of minerals like copper, fluoride and manganese too. Fluoride helps in avoiding cavities in the teeth.

The accumulating scientific data on tea and its constituents — the vitamins, caffeine and tannin - and on its anti-bacterial activity provides a new picture of this popular beverage. Over the past few decades, the list of physiological disorders for which tea is contraindicated has been steadily decreasing. On the other hand, caffeine is sometimes prescribed therapeutically for the treatment of hypertensive headaches and tea is a legitimate means of supplying this medication. Tannin destroys bacteria and virus, thereby inhibiting the growth of dental plaque. But at the same time, tannin inhibits the absorption of iron, calcium and zinc from the food, when tea is consumed along with food.

SUBSTITUTES

- Decaffeinated tea and coffee have their caffeine removed at the green leaves and coffee beans stage. These can be used when caffeine is contraindicated.
- Green tea is better than black tea. It is known to reduce blood pressure, strengthen blood vessels, prevent thrombosis and treat infection.
- Herbal tea has anti-oxidant properties, which lowers the risk of cancer and heart disease.

COFFEE

Coffee arrived in India by sheer accident. A saint of South India, in order to pray, disappeared into a cave in a hillside. His followers kept a vigil outside. It was several months later that the saint emerged from the cave bringing with him seven coffee berries. These he grew on the hills of Karnataka, which are called the 'Baba Budan' hills after him. From this small beginning, coffee plantations spread all over the hilly tracts of the south.

Two types of coffee are grown in our country — 'Arabica and Robusta'. Each has its own flavour and aroma, which are brought out when the beans are roasted and then ground. Roasting was once a home operation, done in a hand turned revolving metal drum over charcoal fire. Today coffee roasting is a commercial exercise. Grinding roasted beans into smaller particles ensures better brew extraction. Brewing is best done in a coffee percolator.

In order to shorten the entire process of making a conventional cup of coffee, instant coffee powders are available — add boiling water, milk and sugar and the coffee is ready. Mixtures of coffee solutes, milk solids and sugar in the form of thick sticky pastes are also being marketed — ready to drink by simply adding boiling water.

In the coffee brew, carbohydrates, proteins and fats are present in very low levels, so the calorie and protein contributions are negligible — they come from the milk added to it.

A cup of coffee clears the mind and abolishes the feeling of fatigue, and can stimulate certain persons even to the point of sleeplessness. It quickens one's reflexes and can aid both mental and physical work. All these qualities stem from caffeine. How? Caffeine (50-80mg/150ml coffee brew) acts on the nervous system, stimulates the lungs, dilates the arteries leading to the heart, and also acts as a diuretic (increasing the urine output). In people suffering from acidity, coffee increases the acid production in the stomach. In healthy people too, over-drinking of coffee may result in acidity so, one is advised to go low on it – maximum 4-6 cups a day.

FOOD ALLERGY

Food allergy has currently become a highly topical subject featuring regularly in the medical journals. Food intolerance or allergy denotes a reproducible clinical reaction to food. It must be distinguished from food aversion, which comprises psychological avoidance and intolerance, where the clinical response does not occur when the food is given in a disguised form.

Food allergies are more common in infants and young children, (0.3-20% of children suffer from symptoms due to food intolerance). Cow's milk protein intolerance, the most common food allergy in childhood has a prevalence between 0.2-7.5%. After the age of five years, there is a tendency to the spontaneous disappearance of the food allergy, while allergy to inhaled substances, such as pollens, dust and animal hairs, becomes increasingly frequent.

The list of foods that have been claimed to cause allergic reactions is very long. It includes such diverse items as eggs, milk, wheat, fish (especially shellfish and other sea foods), various meats, nuts, mustard, tomatoes, oranges and chocolates!

Allergic reactions may affect any system of the body, producing various symptoms. For example, the skin may show a rash, eczema or swollen patches. The respiratory system may be involved in bronchial asthma, sinusitis or bronchitis. The digestive system may show indigestion, vomiting, abdominal pain, diarrhoea and failure of normal growth.

The other allergic symptoms are headache, swelling of joints, conjunctivitis, swelling of lips and tongue, etc.

In some cases of food allergy, the symptoms develop rapidly and dramatically, almost immediately after eating the offending food, and the diagnosis is easy to make. More often, it is not so easy to associate symptoms with any particular food, especially if there is a delay of some hours between the eating of the suspected food and the onset of illness. One has to be very careful in diagnosing the exact allergen - that is, the food responsible for the causation of allergy symptoms.

If the causative food factor is identified, then it can be eliminated from the diet, and the symptoms would not recur. For example, if the responsible article of food is one, which is not consumed regularly (like shellfish), then it can easily be avoided. It is far more difficult in the case of eggs, milk and wheat, which are present in so many foods — cakes, sweets, sauces, soups, biscuits, bread, etc.

Substitution of an alternative food may be possible in the case of milk allergy. A person sensitive to cow's milk may not necessarily be sensitive to goat's milk. Soya bean milk or groundnut milk can also be used as substitutes. Similarly, one sensitive to wheat may do well on oats, rice, barley or corn.

Heating the food may change its properties regarding the causation of allergic symptoms. A person sensitive to raw milk or lightly boiled eggs may be able to tolerate boiled milk or hard-boiled eggs. Many times persons sensitive to eggs are able to take the yolks (yellow part) especially if well cooked, although the egg white continues to cause symptoms.

It is also observed that people tend to outgrow their allergies. Foods known to have caused reactions in childhood may be tried years later with no reactions at all. All people with a well-defined allergy should know about it and inform their doctor. Otherwise they may suffer a severe or even a fatal reaction from a therapeutic injection given for the treatment of some other disease! For instance, a person sensitive to eggs may react badly to immunizing injections prepared on an egg medium, such as those for polio or influenza.

No rigid dietary measures can be established for the treatment of allergic disease. The diet prescription for an allergic person must be specific, individually modified and adjusted, according to the cause of the food allergy, the causative factor naturally being banned from the diet.

FIBRE AND HEALTH

The middle-aged are being afflicted by a plague of modern Western illnesses, many of them being fatal. These illnesses are not caught from germs or viruses – they seem to creep upon us gradually. They are known, collectively, as degenerative diseases, the commonest cause of death in Western countries. The second great destroyer is cancer, cancer of lung, and cancer of bowel being the most common fatal forms of cancer. Apart from these, there is a group of other degenerative diseases like diabetes, diverticulosis and other less serious but still troublesome problems like varicose veins, haemorrhoids and constipation.

The major factor that all these illnesses and health problems have in common is, that they are very rare among the 'third world countries'. Why? It has been found that these communities live on diets which contain a much higher percentage of carbohydrates obtained from cereals which have not been stripped of their dietary fibre, fibre-rich vegetables, legumes and fruits. Such findings have naturally led to a surge of interest in dietary fibre-which for several years was considered to be just one of the unavailable sources of energy in the diet, incidentally having a laxative effect. Dietary fibre is essentially of plant origin. All cereals, fruits and vegetables contain some dietary fibre, but, just as the calorie content of different food varies to a great degree, so does the fibre content. With cereal-based foods, fibre value depends to a large degree on how much has been stripped away in the milling and refining processes. But what exactly is dietary fibre? It can be best described as the carbohydrate material in plant foods that is not digested by man. It is a sponge like material, which absorbs and holds water as it is chewed in the mouth and passes down the gastro-intestinal tract. This means that fibre-rich foods swell to a greater bulk, to fill the stomach, than any other foods.

Dietary fibre is the substance, which makes the waste matter (from the food we eat) pass through us and out of us at a desirable, speedy, natural rate. This is one of the main reasons why it is now considered to be such an important protective factor in saving us from diseases of bowel like cancer. The slow transit rate of fibre-depleted diet is thought to encourage the formation of cancer-forming substances (carcinogens) and other toxins within the body. A high fibre diet would pass through the alimentary canal quickly, giving these carcinogens and toxins very little time to interact in the intestines. The relationship between fibre and constipation is well known. A high fibre diet, thus, relieves a person from constipation and associated problems like haemorrhoids and diverticular disease.

Amongst all the risk factors: cigarette smoking, diet, sedentary living, stress – the strongest for coronary heart disease has been found to be smoking and the strongest protective factor, the intake of cereal fibre. The reason for the beneficial effect of dietary fibre is that it reduces the absorption of cholesterol.

Diabetes involves a faulty insulin production. (Insulin is necessary to control the excess of sugar in the blood). Insulin response to the carbohydrates of the food we eat varies with the speed of absorption of the carbohydrates. Any dietary factor which delays the absorption of carbohydrates may be regarded as beneficial and here once again, dietary fibre appears in a valuable, preventive and protective role. Carbohydrate foods rich in fibre are absorbed more slowly than those from which the fibre has been removed. Hence the popularity of gram flour (high in fibre) in diabetes.

After controlling all the degenerative diseases, fibre goes on to control the body weight too. The principle is simple. Fibre provides no calories, so the total calorie value of a high fibre diet will be less. Secondly, the water absorbing and swelling tendencies of fibre help to fill up the stomach faster and for a longer period of time, thus, the total dietary intake is reduced.

The simplest way to incorporate fibre in the diet is to use more of whole pulses, unseived wheat flour, fresh fruits and vegetables in raw form (not peeling wherever possible) everyday.

METHODS OF COOKING

Pre-historic man was a raw food eater. But gradually he learnt to cook food by direct exposure to flames and by contact with the hot ashes of the hearth. After the clay vessels came into existence, he used them for cooking purpose and found the difference in the taste. Cooking is a refinement that has many advantages and also some hazards in relation to the nutritive value of the food.

Cooking renders the food pleasing to the eye and palate. It also develops a new flavour in the food and stimulates the digestive juices. It facilitates and hastens digestion by altering the texture and makes mastication easier by physical and chemical changes. Cooking sterilizes the food by killing the bacteria and hence improves the keeping quality. It introduces variety. Many different types of dishes can be prepared with the same ingredients.

With all these advantages, cooking however, results in loss of some nutrients depending upon the method used. The various cooking methods are frying, roasting, broiling or grilling, baking, boiling, stewing and steaming.

FRYING

Frying involves cooking the food in hot fat (ghee or oil). It is a quick method and needs continuous careful attention. It can be done by different ways. Sauteing is frying in a small quantity of fat, which is just sufficient to be absorbed by the food cooked in it. Shallow frying is done in a shallow pan like frying pan or skillet using a small amount of fat.

It does not give uniformly good results and is only suitable for either pre-cooked foods like cutlets or foods that need very little cooking like eggs or dosa. Deep-frying is done in a deep saucepan, which contains excess quantity of fat. Food is completely immersed in it. This method gives uniform results and is more economical than shallow frying. Quantity of fat absorbed by the food is very little.

Fried food is delicious to eat and appears to be pleasant looking but at the same time it is difficult to digest. Frying results in loss of vitamins, which can be prevented to some extent by coating the food article with a mixture of plain flour and water, beaten eggs and bread crumbs or just besan batter.

ROASTING

Roasting is cooking over an open fire in a dry medium so that all the surfaces of the food are equally heated. Sometimes, foods like paneer or tender meat are smeared with a little fat before roasting. It is a quick method requiring skill, but some of the vitamins are destroyed as the food comes in direct contact with fire.

BROILING OR GRILLING

It is a very ancient and quick method of cooking. It is cooking by direct dry heat, and high temperature is maintained throughout the cooking time. The food is cooked uncovered. The heat is provided either over or under the food. Only very tender foods can be grilled, like kababs, paneer, tomatoes, mushrooms etc. Since the direct contact with fire is not there, the grilled foods do not lose much vitamins.

BAKING

It is cooking by dry heat in an enclosed vessel or an oven. The enclosed hot air in the oven cooks the food. It is a slow and expensive method of cooking and makes the food very tasty with not much loss in nutrients.

BOILING

It is cooking by moist heat. The food comes in direct contact with boiling water. It is an easy method and does not require constant attention, but the water-soluble vitamins (B and C) are leaked out in the liquid used for boiling. Some flavours may also get lost. Thus, a maximum loss of nutrients takes place in this method. To minimize the losses, the water used for boiling should not be discarded, but used in cooking. Rapid boiling destroys the texture and results in deterioration of nutrients, loss of flavour and makes the food difficult to digest.

STEWING

It is boiling in very small quantity of liquid on a slow heat for a long period of time. It again results in loss of vitamins, especially vitamin C.

BRAISING

It combines two methods, roasting-cum-stewing. The food is first slightly browned in hot fat and then cooked in little water. By doing so there is no loss of nutrients as moisture is entirely used up.

STEAMING

It is also cooking by moist heat, but slower than boiling, unless it is done under pressure. Steamed food is lighter and more easily digestible. The losses of nutrients are minimum. Presssure-cooking is steaming under pressure. It is a better method of cooking since it saves nutrients, fuel and time and makes the food tastier.

NATURE'S PRESCRIPTION FOR COMMON AILMENTS

SKIN DISORDERS

- Steam from strawberry leaves boiled in water on the affected area.
- Instead of soap, pat (not rub) lemon juice on the affected areas. Eat plenty of cabbage, cauliflower and cucumber.
- Drink juice of apple, apricots, kiwi fruits, lemon, raspberries and strawberries. Do a juice fast once a week.
- Avoid alcohol, caffeine, butter, eggs, pineapple, fried foods and sugar.

BRAIN / NERVOUS DISORDERS

- To improve brain function, consume wheat greens, all beans, millets and all nuts.
- Increase the fibre content of your diet.
- Drink juice of apricots, bananas, cherries, grapes, lemons, papaya, peaches, pineapple.
- Avoid cheese, chocolate, corn, eggs, sweets, fats, wheat, fried and processed food.

JOINT DISORDERS

- Avoid spinach, caffeine, all citrus fruits except lemon, eggs, fried foods, salt, fats and sugar.
- Apple and lemons can be combined to give a very healthy juice.
- Grapes, papaya, pears and pineapple are good.

RESPIRATORY DISORDERS

- Avoid whatever (food) provokes attack.
- Certain foods containing sulfites (beetroot, carrot and cold drinks) may provoke an attack.
- Include protein (from cereals, pulses and milk) in the diet for tissue repair.
- Avoid all beans, broccoli, cabbage and cauliflower.
- Apple, grapes, kiwi fruits, lemon, mangoes, papaya and pineapple rarely cause any allergic problems.

HEART DISORDERS

- Wheat germ, soya beans, sunflower seeds should be a part of the diet for all heart disorders.
- Apples, apricots, bananas, grapefruits, lemons, papaya, pomegranates, strawberries, watermelons are excellent fruits for cardiac problems.
- Skins and seeds of red grapes are found to lower the blood cholesterol.
- Brinjal inhibits the rise of blood cholesterol.
- Patients taking blood-thinning medication should avoid broccoli, egg yolk, spinach and cauliflower.
- Olive oil lowers the rate of heart attack.
- Avoid all animal fats, dairy products, fried foods, colas, and hard water.

ULCERS

- Fresh cabbage juice heals ulcers.
- Plenty of water and fibre are important.
- Cabbage, carrot, potatoes, bananas, and papayas are excellent in lowering the acidity.
- Avoid alcohol, caffeine, carbonated drinks, chocolates, fats, fried foods, tobacco and cigarettes.

DIARRHOEA

- Avoid all foods for 24 hours except rice and washed dals.

- Avoid caffeine, fats, nuts and processed foods.
- If persistent, avoid wheat and check for any food allergies.
- Apples, bananas, papayas and peaches can be taken.
- Cooked cabbage and carrot can be taken.

DIABETES

- No fruit juices.
- High complex carbohydrates and high fibre diet is essential.
- Avoid processed foods, fried foods, soft drinks, refined flour, oil capsules.
- Weight control is essential.

FOODS TO STAY YOUNG

AGEING PROCESS

As a person ages, skin cells divide more slowly, and the inner skin, or dermis, starts to thin. Fat cells beneath the dermis begin to atrophy, and the underlying network of elastin and collagen fibres, which provides the foundation for the surface layers, loosens and unravels. Skin loses its elasticity; when pressed, it no longer springs back to its initial position but instead sags and forms furrows.

The skin's ability to retain moisture diminishes; the sweat- and oil-secreting glands atrophy, depriving the skin of their protective water-lipid emulsions. As a consequence, the skin becomes dry and scaly. In addition, the ability of the skin to repair itself diminishes with age, so wounds are slower to heal. Frown lines (those between the eyebrows) and crow's feet (lines that radiate from the corners of the eyes) appear to develop because of permanent small muscle contractions. Habitual facial expressions also form characteristic lines, and gravity accelerates the situation, contributing to the formation of jowls and drooping eyelids.

The skin can also age prematurely as a result of prolonged exposure to ultraviolet radiations from the sun. Other environmental factors, including cigarette smoke and pollution, particularly ozone, may hasten ageing by producing oxygen-free radicals. These are particles produced by many of the body's normal chemical processes. In excessive amounts they can damage cell membranes and interact with genetic material, possibly contributing to the development of a number of skin disorders, including wrinkles and, more importantly, cancer. Rapid weight loss can also cause wrinkles by reducing the volume of fat cells that cushion the face.

The effects of ageing start sooner than we might think. We age along a continuum, rather than all of a sudden. The age-related nutrition issues, from osteoporosis to heart disease, begin in the early adult years.

WE ARE WHAT WE EAT

That means that the foods that we may or may not be eating could be laying the foundation for our health, or lack of it, during our advanced years. Of course, eating well is a difficult choice with the ever-present temptations of fast food and junk food.

But take a look at what these foods are doing to you. Mayonnaise-filled burgers and grease-soaked French fries lead to artery-clogging plaques. And forgoing milk for sugary sodas only encourages the onset of osteoporosis and tooth decay. Add decades of smoking, an inactive lifestyle, stress, and other environmental factors and one will age early and quickly.

The alternate scenario is much more attractive. Minerals from calcium-rich dairy foods and greens can strengthen the bones. Fibre from whole grains helps to keep bowel movements regular. And the antioxidants from fruits and vegetables help prevent cancer from developing by fighting off free radicals, the by-products of the body's everyday processes.

A SIMPLE APPROACH

How do we incorporate more healthy foods into the meals? The easiest way is to add more fruits, vegetables, and whole grains to the daily menu. Most have no fat, cholesterol, or sodium; and they are low in calories. What one gets is lots of fibre, calcium, iron, magnesium, and vitamins, which all play a part in keeping our body functioning at its best.

Researchers are proving it, too. It is reported that people who ate diets high in fruits, vegetables, grains, and white meats were 30% less likely to die of any cause than those who ate red meats, refined cereals and less salads. The conclusion was that heart attacks, osteoporosis, and other signs of ageing take years to develop; and eating healthy foods slows that development.

FOOD FOR OUR SKIN

The skin is the outer reflection of our inner health. Moist, clear, glowing skin is a sign of good diet, while dry, pale, scaly or oily skin results when the diet is not up to par. Fortunately, the eating habits that work best for staying healthy are also the best elixir for our skin.

SKIN TONICS

Just about every nutrient has a role in maintaining healthy skin. Vitamin C helps build collagen, the 'glue' that holds the body's cells together. Poor intake of this vitamin can cause bruising, loss of skin elasticity, poor healing of cuts and scrapes, and dry skin. Just one glass of orange juice or limejuice daily supplies all the vitamin C required. Healthy skin also needs the B-vitamins found in whole grains and milk to help speed wound healing and prevent dry, flaky or oily skin. Vitamin A in red, orange or dark green vegetables and fruits helps prevent premature wrinkling. Zinc in peas, beans and pulses aids in the healing of cuts and scrapes. Water keeps the skin moist and regulates normal function of the oil glands.

GOOD OXYGEN SUPPLY

Our skin needs a constant supply of water and oxygen. Supplying these and other nutrients to the skin and removing waste products requires a healthy blood supply. Nutrients required for building and maintaining healthy red blood cells and other blood factors include protein, iron and copper, plus folic acid, other B vitamins and vitamins C and E. A deficiency of any of these, especially iron, reduces the oxygen-carrying capacity of the blood, suffocating the skin and leaving it pale and drawn.

FATS FOR THE SKIN

Some nutrients directly affect the health of our skin. Repairing damaged skin requires protein, zinc and vitamins A, C and K. Linoleic acid is a fat in vegetable oils that helps restore damaged skin and maintain smooth, moist skin.

ANTIOXIDANTS: ANTI-AGEING AND ANTI-CANCER AGENT

Much of the so-called ageing of the skin is really a result of long-term exposure to sun, pollution and ozone. Environmental pollutants generate highly damaging oxygen fragments, the free radicals that erode skin much like water rusts metal. Free radicals also damage collagen, the protein latticework that maintains the skin's firmness and suppleness. The result is dryness of the skin, loss of elasticity, and the appearance of fine lines and wrinkles.

Free radicals generated by sun exposure also damage the genetic structure of skin cells, which contributes to the development of cancer. Antioxidant nutrients, including vitamins C and E and beta-carotene, slow down the rate of free-radical damage to the skin. People who consume five or more antioxidant-rich foods daily – spinach, sweet potatoes, tomatoes, grapefruit, and carrots – stock these health-enhancing nutrients in their tissues and develop fewer skin cancers.

DIET

The dietary guidelines for healthy, youthful skin are simple. Consume at least 1,200 calories of minimally processed foods daily – including fresh fruits and vegetables, whole grain cereals and pulses, with two to three servings of skimmed milk. Include several servings daily of antioxidant-rich foods, such as citrus fruits for vitamin C, dark green leafy vegetables for beta-carotene, and wheat germ or yeast for vitamin E. Include one linoleic acid-rich food in your daily diet, such as safflower oil.

Drink at least 6 to 8 glasses of water daily. Avoid repeated bouts of weight loss and regain, since weight cycling can result in premature sagging, stretch marks and wrinkling. Take a moderate-dose vitamin and mineral supplement that contains extra amounts of the antioxidant vitamins.

HEALTHY RECIPES

The recipes given below serve two people each. They are easy to cook, using minimal fat and spices and hence, are easy to digest. Weight reduction diets, diabetics, hypertensives, people with painful joints, even ulcers, would benefit from these simple healthy recipes.

MOONG DAL SOUP

½ cup sabut moong dal (preferably sprouted)
1 tsp oil/ghee
1 tbsp tamarind paste
4 cloves garlic, crushed
¼ cup chopped leaves of methi
½ tsp jeera
Salt to taste

Steam dal with chopped methi leaves in 3 cups water for five minutes or till soft. Add tamarind paste and blend in a blender. Add salt to taste. In another saucepan, heat oil, put jeera, when it splutters add crushed garlic. Pour it over the dal, and simmer for 5 minutes.

ANNAPOORNA KARHI

¼ cup arhar dal
2 drumsticks, cut into pieces
4-5 bhindis, cut into pieces
2 tbsp besan
1 tsp oil/ghee
½ tsp each jeera and sarson seeds
¼ tsp haldi

1 tsp dhania powder
Salt and chilli powder to taste
1 tbsp lemon juice

Steam dal with haldi, dhania powder, chilli powder and salt in 4 cups water for 5 minutes. Churn thoroughly. Heat oil and add sarson and jeera seeds. Add besan and fry for 1 minute. Add cooked dal and the cut vegetables. Simmer till the vegetables are soft. Add lemon juice before serving.

PANEER CASSEROLE

¼ kg paneer, cubed
6 cloves garlic, crushed
2 tomatoes and 3 onions, cubed
1 tsp grated ginger
1 small piece pumpkin, cubed
1 cup sprouted moong
2 tbsp cooking corn
1 tbsp cornflour
1 tsp butter
1″ stick cinnamon
1 cup dry breadcrumbs (preferably from brown bread)

Mix all the ingredients, except cornflour, butter and breadcrumbs, in 4-6 cups water and simmer on a slow flame till soft. Roast cornflour lightly in 1 tsp butter and add to the cooked mixture. Pour out this mixture in a baking dish (lined with butter). Sprinkle a thick layer of breadcrumbs on the surface and bake for 15 minutes in a moderately hot oven.

CABBAGE ROLLS

1 medium cabbage
1 cup rice, cooked with a pinch of haldi and salt
1 tsp curry powder
¼ cup boiled peas
Lemon juice to taste

Separate cabbage leaves, keeping them whole as far as possible. Remove any hard core. Soften leaves in hot water for 5 minutes. Grate the inside hard part of the cabbage and mix with the rice, peas and coriander leaves. Add curry powder and lemon juice to taste.

Drain cabbage leaves. Put a little of the mixture in the centre and wrap each leaf around. Arrange in a row, seam side down, in a baking tray. Arrange the remaining stuffing, if any, on either side. Bake for 20 minutes in a moderately hot oven, or steam for 20 minutes.

SAUCY CAULIFLOWER

1 cauliflower (approx. 400 gm) broken into flowerets
1 onion, chopped
1 small piece ginger, grated
2 cloves garlic, crushed
½ cup tomato puree
1 tbsp butter
½ tsp sugar
1 tsp brown vinegar
Salt to taste
(Soya sauce and chilli sauce may be added if desired)

Cook cauliflower with a pinch of salt in just enough water. Arrange in a shallow serving dish. Heat butter and fry onion, garlic and ginger till the onions are soft and transparent. Add tomato puree, vinegar, sugar, salt and simmer for 5 minutes. Pour the sauce all around the cauliflower.

CARROT PARANTHAS

1 cup grated carrot
¾ cup atta
¼ cup besan
¼ tsp jeera powder
A pinch of ajwain

Salt and chilli powder to taste
Oil/ghee for cooking

With oiled fingers, knead all the ingredients into a soft dough, adding water only if necessary. Roll out, as for chapatis. Cook on a tava with very little oil. A non-stick tava may also be used.

GREEN KHANDVI

1 cup besan
½ cup finely chopped spinach leaves
½ cup buttermilk
A pinch of chilli powder
1 cup crumbled paneer
Some chopped coriander leaves
1 tsp oil
¼ tsp sarson seeds
Salt to taste

Mix besan, chilli powder, salt, spinach and buttermilk. Churn or mix thoroughly and pressure cook for 7 minutes. Spread thinly on a greased thali. Sprinkle crumbled paneer and some chopped coriander leaves. Cut into 2" strips and roll up. Heat oil, put in the sarson seeds. When they begin to splutter, pour on the khandvi rolls.

MACARONI LOAF

2 cups grated pumpkin
2 cups fresh breadcrumbs
2 eggs
1 cup boiled macaroni
1 tsp garlic paste
A pinch of garam masala
Salt to taste

Mix all ingredients together. Pack in a greased loaf tin and either bake for 30 minutes in a moderately hot oven or steam for 15 minutes. Cut into slices and serve.

SOYA ROLLS

6 chapatis, made in the usual manner
3 eggs, beaten with salt and pepper to taste
A little oil
1 cup soya granules
6 tsp pudina chutney
½ cup chopped cucumber
½ cup grated mooli
Masala—any, according to taste

Soak soya granules in 1-cup water to swell. Drain, and cook like bhurji, with minimal oil, salt and masala to taste. Dip each chapati in beaten eggs and cook on both sides in a non-stick pan, using very little oil. Apply pudina chutney on each roll and spread some cooked soya stuffing on top. Roll the chapatis and place on a serving dish, seam side down. Arrange chopped cucumber and grated mooli all around.

DHOKLA PIZZA

1 cup moong dal
2 tbsp urad dal
½ cup rice
1 tsp Oil
2 tsp salt
2 tsp yeast granules
2 tbsp. tomato pulp, with salt & pepper to taste
1 small piece cabbage, shredded
1 small capsicum, sliced
100 gm paneer, crumbled

Soak rice and dals in water for 2 hours. Grind the dal-rice mixture to a fine paste. Soak the yeast granules with salt in a little warm water for 5 minutes. Add to the dal mixture and mix it thoroughly. Leave it to ferment for 2 hours. Pour into a greased shallow vessel and top with tomato pulp, shredded cabbage, sliced capsicum and crumbled paneer. Bake in a moderate oven for 25-30 minutes, or steam in a pressure-cooker (as for dhoklas) for 15 minutes.

EGGLESS TOMATO OMELETTE

1 tbsp tomato pulp
1 small onion, finely chopped
1 tbsp grated paneer
Salt and pepper to taste
2 tbsp besan
2 tbsp cornflour
Water as needed (approx. 1 cup)
A little oil

Mix the first four ingredients together and keep aside. Make a smooth batter with cornflour and besan, using just enough water and a pinch of salt. Grease a frying pan with oil and pour in half of the tomato mixture, spreading it a little. Pour half the batter over, allowing it to spread evenly over the tomato. Cook like an uthappam. Make the second omelette in the same way.

STUFFED CAPSICUMS

4 capsicums
½ cup rice
½ cup shelled green peas
1-cup tomato juice
1 tbsp chopped coriander leaves
Salt to taste

Halve the capsicums and remove the seeds. Wash rice well. Cook rice and peas with tomato juice and salt. Mix in coriander leaves. Stuff mixture into the capsicum halves. Steam till capsicums are soft (about 5-7 minutes).